AF572556

DON'T BE AFRAID OF CATARACTS

DON'T BE AFRAID OF CATARACTS

by

DENNIS L. BROOKS, M.D.,
Chairman, Department of Ophthalmology,
Germantown Hospital, Philadelphia

with

ARTHUR HENLEY

Lyle Stuart *Secaucus, N.J.*

To my mother and father, who spent their lives teaching me faith and hope.
And to my children, Dennis and Stephanie, who taught me love and patience.

D.L.B.

Second printing, 1980

Published by Lyle Stuart Inc.
120 Enterprise Ave., Secaucus, N.J. 07094
Published simultaneously by George J. McLeod Limited
73 Bathurst St., Toronto, Ont.
Address queries regarding rights and permissions
to Lyle Stuart Inc.
Manufactured in the United States of America

Library of Congress Cataloging in Publication Data

Brooks, Dennis L
Don't be afraid of cataracts.

Includes index.
1. Cataract. 2. Cataract—Surgery. I. Henley, Arthur, joint author. II. Title.
RE451.B76 617.7'42 78-12696
ISBN 0-8184-0272-5

Contents

DON'T BE AFRAID OF CATARACTS

I

How to Tell if You Have a Cataract

You, or someone you know, cannot see clearly.

The house across the street has a ghostlike appearance. There seems to be a veil over the specials piled high in the supermarket aisle. When you drive at night, the headlights from other cars seem to be more glaring. Street lamps seem to wear halos. You're beginning to rub your eyes when reading the evening paper or watching television. What once appeared to be clear white now seems to be yellow.

The change in your vision is giving you trouble on the job, in the kitchen, when driving, because your eyes just don't seem to focus the way they used to do. Things blur, as when the water runs into your eyes in the shower. And if you wear eyeglasses, you can never seem to get them quite clean enough to see through clearly. It is as if you had rubbed soap over their lenses, smearing them.

But nothing hurts. You have no fever, no headache, no feeling of weakness.

What you do have is a cataract.

It is nothing to be frightened about.

You will not lose your sight. You will see again, just as clearly as you saw before your vision was affected.

Let me tell you what has happened.

The lens in your eye that focuses the light that comes through has become clouded. So less light is coming through.

And the light that is coming through is not being focused clearly on the retina, the "movie screen" in your eye, because of chemical changes in the lens that have affected its ability to focus clearly.

That is all that has happened.

It is not because of something you have done to yourself through poor eating habits, by smoking too much, or by drinking too much.

It is not the result of a disease you have caught or inherited. It is a very natural occurrence that happens usually as a consequence of growing older.

And if it has not already happened to you, only to someone else, it will. Just as it will surely happen to me and to everyone else.

Getting a cataract is like getting gray hair. If you live long enough, you will get both.

Unlike gray hair, however, you cannot make it

disappear or seem to disappear. No drug, no eyedrop, no special kind of diet will cause any kind of change whatsoever.

Resting your eyes will make absolutely no difference.

Getting stronger glasses will make absolutely no difference.

Switching to contact lenses will make absolutely no difference.

But if you do not do something about that cataract, your eye will lose its ability to see anything at all. You will surely go blind, first in one eye, then in the other.

The terrible prospect of blindness is frightening, as it should be. According to a recent Gallup poll, in fact, it is more frightening to most people than any other disability than cancer.

Unlike many cancers, however, all cataracts are curable!

That is the good news, and good news it is, indeed. It means that you need never join those unfortunate individuals whose dread of cataract surgery has left them blind. Or those who postponed cataract surgery to the point at which their nerves became frazzled because they were forced to grope about in semidarkness for so long.

It breaks my heart to see the needless suffering these people have endured because of their misconceptions about cataract surgery.

Do you know that you can have that cataract removed, quickly and painlessly, even in the space of your lunch hour?

Do you know that such an operation is nothing to be afraid of?

Do you know that cataract surgery probably has the highest rate of success of all operative procedures?

If you know these things, then you will know, too, that cataracts are nothing to be afraid of, that "lunch-hour surgery," as it is sometimes called, can eliminate these threats to vision.

In fact, there is very little else in medicine that is so reliable and problem-free as cataract surgery by any method, but especially when done by a procedure called phacoemulsification or "ultrasound," which eliminate or drastically cuts down the need for any hospitalization.

I have used this microsurgical technique and ultrasound procedure on thousands of patients of all ages, both sexes, limiting myself to about 20 such operations a week. In most, I combine the operation for cataract removal with replacement of the clouded lens with a clear new one, an artificial lens implant that will never need replacement.

I am going to tell you more about this technique as well as about the old-fashioned procedure in these pages to help remove your fears of cataract surgery for yourself, a member of your family, or a friend.

It was my good fortune to learn this technique more than a decade ago at the Manhattan Eye, Ear and Throat Hospital in New York City. I felt then that this procedure would revolutionize cataract surgery. My confidence increased when an energetic, peppery woman of 67 came to see me and said, "I have a cataract, and it is making me miserable. I've heard such awful stories about cataract operations that I've kept putting it off. But I heard about this new kind of operation, and I'd like to try it."

Her name—her real name, incidentally—is Carol Dickey, a very active woman whose great love was horses. She loved to ride, and the cataract was making that impossible. She had a terrible fear that she would never be able to ride again and told me, "I just couldn't handle that."

Her fear of not being herself again made her reject the standard cataract operation and instead take her chances on the new ultrasound technique.

I gave her a tranquilizer and then a local eye anesthetic. The operation took fifteen minutes.

When she left the hospital, she took the train back home to downtown Philadelphia. There she changed to a local and walked the rest of the way to her home in Mt. Airy. That same evening, she drove her car to a friend's house, went out to dinner, then drove home again and watched a little television before going to bed.

When she returned to see me for a checkup, she told me, "The train ride home was delightful. I just sat back and watched the scenery go by. I could actually see again. In fact, if I'd had my car with me, I'd have driven directly home. It's a terrific operation. I feel like I'm living again."

Within a week, she was able to ride horseback again. That was her greatest joy.

As her doctor, it was also my great pleasure to

see her able to resume her normal activities. For I do not consider my job as an ophthalmologist merely one that enables a patient to read more letters on an eye chart. That alone will not make life more pleasant. Getting rid of a cataract is only one step in the process of seeing again. After removing a cataract, you have to regain the vision you need to live better, do your work efficiently, and give up feeling like an invalid.

If you are reading this book because someone you know has a cataract, but you do not, try this little experiment. Take a drinking class with a flat bottom and rub a bit of soap on the bottom. gnvow look through it. That is how things might look when you have a cataract.

Soapy.

But there is no film covering that lens in your eye that can be scrubbed off like the soap on your drinking glass. The "soapiness" goes through and through the entire lens.

To be able to see again, the entire lens must be removed and replaced either by a new artificial lens, cataract glasses, or a contact lens in order for you to see again like your old self. The information you need to make that choice will be dealt with in another chapter of this book.

What you should know at the outset is that cataract surgery itself is not new. What is new and different is the ultrasound technique based on the principle of phacoemulsification. "Phaco" is a Greek word for "lens," and emulsification means only that a solid substance is reduced to a liquid.

The phacoemulsification procedure is nothing more than that: reducing that solid blurry lens to a liquid.

It is done with microsurgery, which means that the ophthalmologist must operate while peering through a high-power microscope. Using this technique, a single stitch that soon after dissolves harmlessly is all that is necessary.

This is quite unlike the standard "old-fashioned" procedure, feared by Carol Dickey, which requires some 8–10 stitches, all of which usually have to be removed, as well as many days of hospitalization. The recuperative period can, in fact, stretch out to several months.

But even the old-fashioned method cures cataracts.

That is why my chief concern here is to help you banish your fears about cataract surgery. With today's technology, there is no reason to put off the operation.

I agree with those of my professional colleagues who feel that a cataract surgeon should be able to do all types of cataract operations. My preference is for the ultrasound procedure, but if I encounter the unusual situation in which that procedure is unsuitable, I refine that procedure, alter part of the technique, and, if necessary, confine myself to the conventional procedure or some variation of it.

But this has nothing to do with the implantation of an artificial lens, only with the removal of the cataract. Unlike the traditional method of inserting a new lens, often done—and I find this truly astonishing—without the use of a microscope, I employ only fine microsurgical techniques.

Moreover, an artificial lens implanted in the standard, old-fashioned way is supported in the eye only by the iris and the vitreous, a jellylike substance, and this does not offer very firm support.

I always leave intact in the eye that part that held the original but clouded lens in place. The back part of that capsule, as it is called, stays in the eye to hold the new artificial replacement lens tightly, permanently, like a fine pocket watch held firmly in its perfectly fitted case. This approach is far less disturbing to the eye, and that means less discomfort to you, the patient.

Let me dip into my patient file again and tell you about a lovely lady, Mrs. Anna Harple, who had an absolute dread of cataract surgery and a great reluctance to use either cataract eyeglasses or contact lenses.

"My world is a fuzzy mess," she told me. "I know I have cataracts in both eyes. But I've been hoping and praying that they'd get better by themselves. Instead, they've gotten worse and worse. I can't read a recipe anymore. I can't even see across the street. Now I know that something has to be done, and, frankly, I'm scared stiff."

"Why are you so frightened?" I asked her.

"Because I can never forget what my father went through when he had cataracts," she replied. "He was in the hospital for ten days and then had to stay out of work for three months. On top of that, he had to wear thick lenses to be able to see again. That's not for me."

I reassured her that such an ordeal was no longer necessary. She agreed to let me remove the cataracts by ultrasound and replace them with artificial lenses.

I did one eye at a time, each time using a two-step procedure. The first step was to transform the old lens painlessly into jelly with ultrasound and just as painlessly draw out that jellied lens. The second step, immediately following the first, was to slip in the new lens. I did the second eye exactly the same way three months later.

Her vision in both eyes, which was perfect before the onset of the cataracts, was restored again to what it was originally: 20/20, with normal side vision as well.

I am often asked why an eye operation of any kind puts so much fear into most people. In Mrs. Harple's case, it was due in great part to her father's bad experience. In the other case, concerning Miss Dickey, it was due to her worry that cataract surgery would leave her too restricted to enjoy her customary life style.

But I think there is more to this fear, and it has to do with our psychological attitudes. To most of us, seeing is something magical.

This magical power is evident in the old wives' tales about "the evil eye" and the ability of its possessor to wreak havoc on anyone with a mere glance.

On the other hand, the gift of sight makes it possible for us to maintain our guard against whatever would harm us, to be vigilant, watchful, perceptive. "Keep an eye on that scoundrel," we're warned. And there are countless similar admonitions: "Keep an eye on your luggage" and "on your pocketbook" and "on your child."

In other words, it is our eyes that take up guard duty not only for our bodies but for those we love and for our prized possessions. And these eyes of ours are vulnerable, protected only by seemingly delicate eyelids, lashes, and a blink to act as a shield.

So in addition to being a source of enjoyment as our "windows to the world," our eyes serve also as a means of protecting ourselves, warding off evil.

As a consequence, the very thought of anything, from an eyedrop to a surgeon's fine instrument held in skillful hands, is likely to be quite threatening. This feeling has been reinforced by historical, literary, and everyday stories.

How many times did you read in your school books about victorious warriors "gouging out" or "plucking out" the eyeballs of their victims?

How often were you reminded by a well-intentioned, concerned parent to be careful not to "poke your eyes out" when at play?

And by now everyone is familiar with the Oedipus complex put forth by Dr. Sigmund Freud in his psychoanalytical writings based on young Oedipus, the hero of classical literature, who was deprived of his sight for even thinking the unthinkable thought of sleeping with his mother.

All of these references have become part of our unconscious mind, lingering on to reinforce our very natural fears of losing the use of our eyes and becoming blind.

But while the gift of sight is probably valued more highly than all our other senses, it is somehow the one most taken for granted, until it begins to fail. And that is when all those unconscious remembrances surface.

When we are actually threatened by the loss of sight, we become startingly aware of its value and begin to feel more strongly the terror of not being able to see again.

And, yes, even though you may find this hard to believe, I have learned from my experience as an ophthalmologist that many people feel a sense of shame upon learning that cataracts are responsible for robbing them of sight. They blame themselves.

I sometimes feel it is their way of compensating for their true fear of becoming blind and dependent.

Foolish? Of course!

If you get a cataract, it is not your fault. I am going to show you how it can happen to anyone, at any age, and how it can be gotten rid of.

Without fear.

II

Cataracts Happen at Any Age

Doctors are a funny bunch. For reasons that I never could understand, they like to speak in a language that their patients do not understand.

For example, there are eye specialists who have examined a patient and then said, "You have a progressive lenticular opacity in the lens of your eye."

What he really was saying was "You have a cataract."

He did not put it that way because he thought it might be more frightening, or perhaps because he thought it might seem more professional to express the diagnosis in scientific language.

But I think scientific jargon is more frightening to patients than ordinary talk. This often means more than simply telling someone, "You have a cataract."

It means saying what it is, what it is not, and what it means. Simple language that everybody understands is to me the first step in eliminating fear.

In this book, I am going to talk to you as if you were my patient, coming to me with complaints about disturbing symptoms that interfere with your vision and in whom I have diagnosed the formation of a cataract.

And the first thing I will tell you after that is that you do not have any eye disease. All that you have is a visual impairment that can very easily be corrected.

The second thing I will tell you is that you have a lot of company. At least 3 million men and women like you have the same problem, and at least a half million of these will have cataract surgery before the year is over. In fact, three out of four eye operations will be for cataracts.

The third thing I will tell you is that two out of three cataract operations are for what are commonly called "senile" cataracts. And I will be quick to advise you, and reassure you, that the word "senile" is really misleading. It has nothing to do with your age. It only means that the lens in your eye has aged, perhaps before its time. A better word to describe it would be "senescent." In short, you have nothing more than a slow-growing cataract that has not grown as slowly as you would have liked.

Let me repeat. There is no connection whatever between the word "senile" as applied to cataracts and to the state of your mind, your intellect, your mental factors. Yet this is the word most commonly used to describe 90 percent of all cataracts, regardless of the age at which they occur.

No one knows precisely why the lens in one person's eye clouds over sooner than it does in another person's eye. It is thought that it might have something to do with the lens, for one reason or another, not getting the kind of nourishment it nees to keep the cells that make up the lens working efficiently.

But this sort of information is really unimportant since we do not yet know enough about the cause to recommend preventive measures. What is important is that we do have enough expertise to eliminate those clouded lenses that trouble you.

Ordinarily, when patients come to see me, they know they have cataracts. As their vision worsened, they suspected it. A relative or friend who had an experience with cataracts suggested this might be the problem. Other doctors often told them so as well, but they kept shopping around for one who would disagree. So great was their fear.

When I talk to them, I learn very quickly to what degree they are handicapped by failing vision. When I examine their eyes through optical instruments, called an ophthalmoscope and slit-lamp biomicroscope, I can see deep inside the eye and determine how far the cataract has progressed. I will also get a clear picture of the general health of the eye, its various parts, and its blood vessels.

On these scientific findings, I can base a firm diagnosis and decide what should be done, how it should be done, and when it should be done. I have to take into consideration not only the extent of the cataract's development but also the general health of the eye and recommend what my patient would be happiest with after surgery: a lens implant, contact lenses, or cataract glasses.

To make such a recommendation, a purely medical decision is not enough. My patient must take part in that decision. Would he or she find cataract glasses too cumbersome or unfashionable, contact lenses too difficult or bothersome to handle, or an implant too fearsome to contemplate despite its great advantage of permanence?

All cataract patients are not alike.

On the one extreme, there is the individual who wants to know absolutely nothing about anything. He or she says only, "Make me see, doctor, however you think best."

On the other extreme, there is the individual who wants to know everything. He or she comes in with a sheaf of statistics and medical articles and asks question after question: "Will I really get back 20/20 vision? How long will my eye take to heal? What will driving be like?"

To such a patient, I make it a point to give very

specific answers, just as I will be doing in this book. Moreover, in this preoperative discussion, I insist on having another member of the family present. It helps for the whole family to know what procedure will be followed once a definitive diagnosis has been made.

I can not stress too strongly the importance of dealing with a patient's personal feelings about an eye operation. This became clear to me years ago at the start of my medical career. My first choice then had been psychiatry, and my training taught me that the mind and body work together, that before contemplating any kind of surgery, a person has to work through his or her fears about such surgery.

Once this has been accomplished and the operation performed, the mind again works with the body to expedite the healing process. No one knows this better than the plastic surgeon, who takes pains to understand a patient's emotional state of mind, the nature of his or her personality, before undertaking a face lift or whatever.

I think it is even more important when it comes to operating on the eye for the reasons pointed out in the previous chapter.

At this point, you may wonder why I changed my specialty from psychiatry to ophthalmology. I did so because I have the good fortune to possess what in the surgical profession is known as "good hands." My fingers have the agility needed for delicate surgical procedures. Besides, I have a great need to see reproducible results. The psychiatrist's cure is not as precise as the surgeon's, not because of a lack of ability but because of the nature of the medical problem.

When I remove a cataract lens from an eye, I know that there are sure-handed ways to do so. I know exactly how the eye is constructed, where I may encounter problems, if any, and how to deal with them. And it gives me great satisfaction to repeat this procedure in patient after patient, eye after eye after eye.

Without becoming too involved, let me tell you something about your eyes and why they are vulnerable to cataracts.

The very front of your eye is a tough but sensitive dome-shaped shield called the cornea. It is the first part of your eye to receive light and commence the process of seeing. Behind it is the iris, which works like a camera shutter, opening and closing in split seconds to alter the amount of light entering the eye.

Behind the iris, in the eye's pupil—the central part of the iris—is the lens. Behind the lens is a jellylike substance called the vitreous, and behind that is the retina, the movie screen of the eye, which receives all the images passing through the lens.

That is the troublemaker, the lens. That is the source of the cataract.

In the normal eye, the lens is clear, like unblemished glass. Light passes through it unobstructed, and whatever is revealed by that light is projected onto the retina. The retina then translates these visual impressions into nerve impulses that are carried to the brain by the optic nerves.

That is how you see.

But if any part of this chain is broken, you cannot see clearly or at all. And the part of the chain most likely to be broken is the lens. Over a period of time, it becomes hardened, less flexible, and cloudy. When that happens, any images that come through it become distorted.

When that happens, you have a cataract.

That lens, in youth, can quickly change its focus to accommodate distant objects and those up close. With time, however, the lens loses more and more of that ability. If you're one of the lucky ones, it may not happen until you're way past retirement age. If you are not so lucky, it can happen at middle age or even sooner. It can also happen at birth or as the result of an accident to your eye, but these are very special kinds of cataracts, which I will deal with later.

What I think you need to know most of all is how this cataract, which ruins your vision, can be extracted no matter what your age.

Do you think 90 is too old for cataract surgery?

Well, if you do, I will tell you about a man named Jesse Yoder who will not agree. When he came to see me at Germantown Hospital in Philadelphia, he said, "Don't be deceived by my age, Dr. Brooks. I'm an active man, and I want to remain active. It means everything to me to have my vision back."

Mr. Yoder loved to read, to drive. He enjoyed

traveling. He enjoyed reading the fine books in his home. He did not see himself as a victim of old age but merely as a victim of a cataract.

It was not his first cataract. Many years before, he had a cataract removed from one eye by the old-fashioned method, and he was able to see well through that eye. But he could not see well enough with one eye to do all the things he wanted to do, and he did not want to go through the lengthy procedure he had experienced before.

I scheduled the ultrasound operation for noon. It required no more than 15 minutes. He then made himself comfortable in my office until the tranquilizer wore off. And by two o'clock that same afternoon, he was on his way home. There was no need for a single night's hospitalization.

"I was in by noon, out by two," he told me happily. "I find it remarkable. My vision's good again. I can read all I want to with both eyes, and my eyes don't get tired. I'm also able to drive my car more confidently, and that means a lot to a man of my age."

For Mr. Yoder, I prescribed cataract glasses because contact lenses would be too much of a bother for him, and since he had already had a cataract removed from the other eye by standard surgery, there was no reason to implant an artificial lens in the second eye. Moreover, he found cataract glasses perfect for his needs, which proves what I said earlier about the need to come to a mutual decision in the patient-doctor relationship.

All right, so now I have told you about an elderly man who suffered from a cataract. But I have also made clear that one's age is not a true determinant of cataract development.

Are you middle-aged and bothered by a cataract? And are you wondering, "How can this happen to me? I'm not old enough to get a cataract?"

But that is the way of cataracts. They are not necessarily respecters of one's chronological age.

I am again going to dip into my patient file and tell you about a gentleman named Stanley Wallace. Only middle-aged, he was plagued by cataracts in both eyes, and he was terrified at the prospect of undergoing eye surgery. It was his wife who convinced him that he should do something about them if he hoped to continue working.

"I've heard so many nightmarish stories about cataract operations," he told me, "that, frankly, I'm scared to death."

I used a bit of psychology on him. I did not make any reply to his statement but instead asked him to please take a seat in my waiting room. I wanted him and his wife to have the opportunity to talk with other patients.

When I called him back into my office, he said, "You know, I'm beginning to feel better about having the operation. I've been talking to your other patients, and I can't get over it—they're all full of smiles and nobody seems to be afraid."

My psychology had worked. This was a patient who needed support from other patients who had been through the kind of surgery he dreaded so much. They did better at relieving his anxieties than I could have done myself.

Both he and his wife agreed that I should operate on both eyes. We agreed, too, that he would be most comfortable with contact lenses after surgery. He did not want to be bothered with cataract glasses and did not want lens implants.

Fine. But was he sure that contact lenses would be agreeable and easy to handle?

After explaining to him the kind of care and attention contact lenses required, he assured me that they would do fine and that he would prefer them. My examination of his eyes confirmed the fact that he could use them quite well.

Using ultrasound, I performed the necessary operations on both eyes only a few days apart, for there were no complications, no difficulties. And later I fitted him with the contact lenses he desired.

Right after the operation, he said to me, "I feel no pain at all."

A day later, he said, "My eyes feel just fine, and I can see again."

After I fitted him with contact lenses, he said, "I can see perfectly now. I feel just like a young man again. I can actually go back to work right away."

So there you have documented examples of so-called "senile" cataracts occurring at ages almost half a century apart. And I think it is important that you understand this because it has a lot to do with the way you feel about yourself just as much as it has to do with your concern about your vision.

I hope that readers of this book will know by now that cataracts are not tumors, not infections, and not the result of some individual shortcoming.

In almost all cases, they are no more than natural consequences of living. That is all. But there are some exceptions, of course. Aside from the possibility of congenital formation or the result of trauma (injury) to the eye, cataracts could be secondary to other kinds of eye disease.

The late Elvis Presley, for example, was said to have suffered from an inflammatory eye disease called uveitis that could cause a disturbance in the eye that would lead to the formation of a cataract. If this had eventuated, it would be termed a secondary cataract, meaning that it was triggered by another eye problem and not full grown by itself.

Also, there are problems evolving from glaucoma, diabetes, and hypertension that influence the growth and treatment of cataracts, but these are minor when compared to the great majority of cataracts. Nevertheless, I will deal with these kinds of cataracts later in this book.

What I consider paramount is for all readers to feel secure about the professional expertise currently available to treat all kinds of cataracts no matter what their source may be. And in almost all situations, these cataracts will be what are called primary, simple and unrelated to any hereditary problem, accident, or eye disease.

Thus, there is only one question to be answered, and that is: when to have that cataract removed so that full sight can be restored.

III

When to Do Something About Cataracts

One of the most common misconceptions about cataracts is that they have to be "ripe" before they can be removed.

Ripe?

Like grapes? Tomatoes? Cantaloupes?

After anything ripens, it quickly progresses to where it becomes overripe, and finally it rots. Just as rotted fruit can do mischief to the digestive system, rotted cataracts can do mischief to the eye.

I would like to spend a little time discussing this because it is probably the most frequent question raised by cataract patients. But before expressing my own views on the subject, I want to quote a statement made by the highly respectable American Association of Ophthalmology:

> Cataract surgery, which has a high rate of success, need not be postponed until the cataract is "ripe." Surgery should be considered when a cataract has progressed to the point that it interferes with a person's ability to function satisfactorily and when glasses are no longer able to provide sufficient visual improvement.

The average eye doctor uses the word "ripe" as an excuse to postpone operating on the bad eye until vision in the other eye becomes equally poor. He tells the patient, "You have to wait. Your cataract isn't ripe enough."

What he really means is that the cataract developing in the good eye has not progressed enough to warrant surgery in the bad eye.

If this sounds ridiculous, it is. More than that, it is heartbreaking. I see men and women every day who have sat around for months, even years, waiting for the "ripe" moment while their lives have gone to pieces because their vision has deteriorated. The bad eye has worsened, and the good eye has worsened, too. The loss of vision has made that person befuddled, depressed, and more fearful than ever.

Why, then, would a thoroughly capable eye specialist put off cataract surgery?

For one thing, he does not do implant surgery. If he did, he could immediately remove the cataract from the bad eye and replace it with an intraocular lens, an artificial lens implant. This would restore full vision to the bad eye and allow full use of both eyes. The other eye could then be operated on when it also commences to lose vision due to the progression of the cataract clouding that eye.

Even if he does not do implant surgery, he could operate immediately on the bad eye and make it see again with a contact lens. But very likely he knows that the patient he is dealing with is not the sort who will be able to handle a contact lens.

That could present another problem if the doctor uses the old-fashioned procedure to remove the cataract from the bad eye. With that procedure, there is a long recovery process. Without a lens implant or contact lens, that patient would have to wear cataract glasses, and these could not be used if only one eye is operated on.

I will talk about this problem in greater detail later. For now, let me just say that the high-powered lenses in cataract glasses magnify images greatly, so greatly that you would see a far larger image through one eye than the other. The result would be double vision, and that would be unbearable.

What I want to make clear in this chapter is that there is no need—in fact, it would be sheer folly—to wait until both eyes have become overwhelmed by cataracts.

But do not take just my word for it. Listen to what a man named Ted Hoeger, better known as Captain Tate to patrons of his seafood restaurant on the South Jersey shore, told me when he came to my office.

"I'm a nervous wreck," he said. "My business is suffering, and I'm suffering. I can't drive my car without cracking it up. I take hours and hours to read a newspaper with the most powerful magnifying glass I could buy. And it's all because of these miserable cataracts.

"They began to bother me years ago but my doctor kept telling me to wait, wait, wait, they weren't ripe enough to operate. I've been sitting around waiting more than two years. Now I've had to come to see you like a blind man holding on to my wife's arm!"

Two years of this man's life had gone to waste. It was shameful. Aside from his inability to see, he was a healthy man. I was able to treat him as an outpatient and send him home the same day.

Quite literally, he could not believe his eyes. He elected to have contact lenses and told me, "Everything is beautiful, and business is booming."

Mrs. Hoeger, who also had cataracts, and who had also been told to wait because both eyes were not equally affected, decided to have the worse eye operated on immediately. She elected to have a lens implant. It made her husband a little bit jealous because she will never have to bother with contact lenses or cataract glasses.

I do not want to burden you with medical jargon, but there are some things about cataracts that you should know because you may have come across these terms in your reading or perhaps have heard them mentioned somewhere.

One such term is "incipient." It is a way of describing an early cataract that is not bothering your vision too much. There is not much blur, there is not much fuzziness, there is not much yellowing. Things just do not seem quite as clear as they once did.

Another term used frequently is "immature." It means almost the same as "incipient." Your vision is not really too bad. You can see well enough to do just about everything you always do.

"Mature" is what many doctors call a cataract they classify as "ripe." But because the word "ripe" often means different things to different eye doctors, as I have just explained, I prefer the term "mature." What it means to me is that your cataract has progressed to a point where it most definitely is interfering with the way you see and, as a result, is making your life much more difficult. Its progression has reached the point where cataract surgery is indicated.

Now let us take a giant step. If your cataract is characterized as "hypermature," you have let it go far too long. Your eye is in danger of becoming very inflamed and is very possibly causing sufficient pressure on the optic nerve to lead to glaucoma. The risk of that cataractous lens rupturing is very real.

At that stage, the lens may have become so swollen that it has turned white. You may be able to see light or perhaps even vague shapes moving in front of you—hand motions, they are called—but the condition is tantamount to blindness.

The cataract may even be visible to others, not just an eye doctor, because the pupil is no longer black. When a light is shined on it, the pupil appears white because whoever is looking at it is, in fact, looking through it directly at the cataract. At this late stage, an emergency operation is necessary to save the eye.

That is why I urge you not to put off cataract surgery in the wild hope that your clouded lens will clear up by itself in time. While it is true that some cataracts progress more slowly than others, it is also true that they do progress.

Now I am sure that some of you readers are saying to yourselves, "Ah, that doctor is forgetting something called 'second sight' where suddenly you start to see better all over again without any kind of treatment at all!"

Well, I have not forgotten about the phenomenon called "second sight," but it is going to come as a surprise to a lot of you to know what it really means.

It means that a cataract is forming in your eye.

Let us assume, for example, that you are farsighted. You do not have any need for eyeglasses for distant viewing. At the age of forty or so, you find that you do require glasses for reading but still not for distance. After a while, perhaps years later, you notice something strange happening. You no longer need reading glasses. And you say to yourself, "Isn't this wonderful? My eyes have gotten better. I can read perfectly well again without glasses."

Do you know what has happened?

You have become nearsighted because there are changes going on in the lens in your eye. If you had been visiting the same eye doctor over a period of time for regular eye checkups, he would have noticed the change in your sight. He would have noted the changes he made in your eyeglass prescription over the years.

Eyeglass power is measured in something called diopters. Your regular eye doctor will note that you have gone from, say, two diopters farsighted to one diopter farsighted and the next year have not required any corrective lenses at all, but the following year, one diopter nearsighted, then two diopters nearsighted, and so on.

If you had visited different eye doctors or optometrists, there would be no record of such changes. Only you would be in a position to notice such changes.

That is the meaning of the term "second sight." It does not mean that you had a cataract that is getting better by itself. On the contrary, it means that you have a clue to the fact that a cataract is forming.

But let me make it clear that it is not a symptom to cause you worry. You do not have a cataract of a kind that demands immediate attention. It may take many years before the cataract forms to the degree to which it requires removal.

If I seem to belabor this point, it is only because I want to rid you of the misconception that the phenomenon of "second sight" is a sign that a cataract is disappearing of itself.

The real symptoms of cataracts are obvious.

Less light enters your eye. Your vision dims. You may see ghostlike images. Things are not clear. When you look at a bright light, you may see halos around the source of that light, a frequent occurrence while driving at night. Everything may appear more yellow in color. Little by little, there is an increasing blurriness in everything that meets your eye, whether it be up close or at a distance. And you may see peculiar spots that remain stationary, not moving about, especially when looking at some particularly bright image.

The younger you are, the more rapidly that cataract tends to develop. Sometimes it happens unbelievably fast, even within a few months. I am talking about men and women in their forties or even fifties.

But the older you are, the more slowly that cataract generally progresses. This is why many elderly people tend to postpone cataract surgery until they become nearly blind.

The reason for this discrepancy is that not all cataracts are the same. Younger people most often have what are called posterior subcapsular cataracts in which the entire lens is fairly clear except for the back part. Among older people, nuclear cataracts are more common, and the heart of the lens is affected.

In my practice, I often meet with the grown children of elderly people before meeting the patient himself, or herself, as the case may be. For the children are very confused about their parent's failing sight. It is causing trouble not only to the parent but to the children as well. They are fearful of allowing the parent to go out alone. They brood over the parent's inability to find amusement in reading or watching television. Yet they worry that the patient's age might be a barrier to surgery.

I will tell you right now that few, if any, elderly citizens are too old for ultrasound removal of cataracts. Later on in this book, I will go into more detail about special considerations for special situations. But such special situations affect only a small minority of individuals.

Nevertheless, it sometimes requires an inordinate degree of motivation to get an aging parent to agree to cataract surgery, so great is their fear—and sometimes the fear of their children as well.

Let me give you an example. Mr. Joseph B. Van Sciver, Jr., was 81 years old when he visited my office. Through one eye, he could barely see light and had been diagnosed as "hopelessly blind" and "inoperable" by specialists at two leading eye hospitals because he suffered also from hardening of the arteries.

The old-fashioned standard operation for cataracts would have required a lengthy stay in the hospital that would keep him in bed for many days. This could lead to complications for a man with arterial problems. The ultrasound technique, however, made such long bed rest unnecessary.

In view of the advice given him and his children, Mr. Van Sciver kept putting off surgery. But it troubled him greatly that he had never seen his grandchildren, for he was functionally blind. He was able to speak with them, touch them, but could not distinguish them in the blur that stole away his sight.

This was the motivation that brought him to me, to learn if perhaps my procedure could restore his sight.

After carefully examining his eyes and taking into consideration the whole state of his physical health, I felt that I could safely reassure him that I could operate, doing one eye at a time.

There was no problem with the surgery. In view of his age and his other medical problem, however, I insisted that he remain overnight at the hospital.

The following day he went home, on the arm of his grandchild, whom he was able to see for the first time in his life. Not very clearly, of course, but clearly enough to make out her features.

Before a month had gone by, Mr. Van Sciver had gotten back—and this amazed even me—20/20 vision in that operated eye with the aid of cataract glasses. I was able to prescribe such glasses because he could not see at all with the other eye; hence, there was no problem of his experiencing double vision.

He was ecstatic about actually being able to see his grandchildren at last. He finally felt like a full-fledged grandfather.

Still, I must confess that I was a little disappointed. I wanted to operate on the other eye as well. But Mr. Van Sciver, so long accustomed to having no sight at all, told me, "No, thank you, Dr. Brooks. I already have perfect sight in one eye. That's more than I've had since I can remember, and, at my age, I think that's enough."

For some people, though, it is not enough. Take someone for whom anything less than perfect vision in both eyes can be a catastrophe.

An airline pilot is a perfect case in point. His vision must be flawless. And if it is obstructed to even a small degree by cataracts that formed while he was still young enough to fly commercially, he would have to undergo cataract surgery to retrieve that perfect vision.

And that is quite possible. Vision can be refined just that tiny bit needed to enable someone like an airline pilot to keep his job.

I will tell you more about this aspect later, and also about congenital cataracts that afflict some children at birth. If a child has a cataract in one eye, it must be corrected before the age of 6 because that child's brain is not sending the kinds of messages necessary for use of that eye, and so the eye with the cataract is not being used. It becomes what we call a "lazy eye," or, in medical language, a condition known as amblyopia. And if that cataract is not removed before the age of 6, the child will never be able to see well.

But it is just as safe to do cataract surgery on a child as it is to do it on an adult of any age. The decision is not whether or not it should be done but how it should be done.

IV

What to Do About Cataracts

There is more than one way to remove a cataract safely. One is by conventional surgery, a procedure I have referred to in this book as the old-fashioned method. The other is by phacoemulsification surgery, a procedure I have referred to as the ultrasound method. Both methods are effective, but the ultrasound technique offers the cataract patient many advantages in terms of the operation itself as well as in the healing process that follows, most particularly when the patient desires to have the cataract replaced with an artificial lens implant.

I am going to explain both procedures and compare them side by side so that you will have a better understanding of just what happens during a cataract operation.

However, I would first like to mention a Biblical saying with which all of you are familiar: "An eye for an eye, and a tooth for a tooth."

What does that have to do with cataract surgery?

Everything.

The ultrasound instrument that dissolves your cataract works very much like the modern dental drill that dissolves the decay in a bad tooth. In both instruments, high-frequency sound waves vibrate away what must be gotten rid of: the hardened tooth decay and the hardened, cloudy cataract lens.

You know that when an operatic tenor or soprano reaches a high note, he or she can actually cause a glass to shatter. It happens because the vibrations set off by that high-frequency sound are so intense.

Well, the vibrations set off by the ultrasound instrument are even more intense: 40,000 cycles per second. It is so high a sound that it is beyond the range of human hearing. You hear absolutely nothing. And you feel absolutely nothing. Yet it is that sound, ultrasound, that is replacing the surgeon's knife and vibrating your cataract into minute particles that have the consistency of mushy jelly. And that jelly, which was your cataract, is then whisked out of your eye in its emulsified state through a miniaturized hollow tube. And all of this happens in a flash.

That is the essence of the ultrasound method.

And before comparing the full surgical procedure with the old-fashioned operation, it is important that you have some familiarity with the basic ultrasound technique.

In the decade that I have worked with this procedure, I have dedicated myself to perfecting this approach to cataract surgery and combining it with a method of lens implantation that reduces the possibility of any complications to practically zero.

Nevertheless, I want to make something clear right here. Although the ultrasound method is often touted in the press as a kind of miracle cure, neither I nor my colleagues have any pretensions to being "miracle" workers.

We are serious physicians.

What makes the technique work is plain and simple medical technology and expertise. For these reasons, and only these reasons, am I convinced that the ultrasound method does the most to help people overcome their totally unwarranted fears of cataract surgery.

Why do I believe so strongly in its benefits?

Well, let us examine the two procedures—the traditional or conventional one, which I call the old-fashioned way, and the newer ultrasound method—to see how they differ when compared side by side.

In both procedures, the preparation of the patient is virtually identical, with one exception. Before traditional surgery, the patient is given medication called an enzyme to loosen the ligaments in the eye that hold fast the capsule containing the lens clouded by the cataract. This is unnecessary in ultrasound surgery because that part of the capsule held fast by those ligaments is left undisturbed.

Now picture yourself as the patient. Here is what happens to prepare you for either procedure:

1. You are given a simple tranquilizer to relax you.
2. A local anesthetic is administered by injection, quite painlessly, to deaden the nerves and muscles that control your eye and eyelids and to prevent you from blinking or feeling any pain during the operation.
3. Drops are put into your eye to dilate the pupil—make it larger—no differently than what is done in a normal eye examination.
4. The upper and lower eyelids are drawn back.

So far, then, the preparation for the operation is the same for both procedures. But I want to explain why there is no need to loosen those ligaments in the ultrasound operation.

I want those ligaments. They are there for a reason, to help support certain structures in the eye. When they are torn loose, even with the help of medication, it causes a lot of debris to be scattered inside your eye. That could lead to problems afterward. Postoperative glaucoma, for example. It may only be temporary and disappear with treatment, but I prefer to keep things simple, uncomplicated.

For this reason, I very carefully examine my patient's eye in my office before even contemplating surgery. I tap it to see if the lens—that clouded cataract lens—jiggles, because that tells me something about the condition of those ligaments. If they are firm, holding fast, and there is no jiggling, I want them to stay that way. But if those ligaments are weak, not holding, then I will not elect to do ultrasound surgery. I will be forced to use the traditional technique.

It is a rare situation, however, that those ligaments, perhaps due to injury or premature aging, are weak. So it is rarely that I have the need to forsake the ultrasound procedure in favor of the traditional one.

Now let us get back to comparing the two procedures. You are lying down comfortably on the operating table, perhaps enjoying what is sometimes called "twilight sleep," with only your eye exposed. And here is where there is a world of difference between the two procedures.

Both procedures remove cataracts successfully.

The Old-Fashioned Way	*The Ultrasound Way*
1. Most surgeons use a 2- or 3-power magnifier (some use none at all) to view the eye throughout the operation.	1. All surgeons use a special 8- to 20-power microscope to view the eye throughout the operation—far greater magnification.
2. An incision approximately 3/4″ long is made in the eye. It is about the width of your thumbnail and extends nearly halfway around the eyeball.	2. An incision about 1/16″ wide is made. That is little more than the thickness of a single wire of a paper clip, and that is plenty wide enough.
3. The cornea, the outer coating of the eye, is lifted slightly away from the eye and held out of the way with a clamp to make the eye accessible to surgery.	3. Using the operating microscope, the surgeon inserts the hollow tiny tip of the ultrasound probe through the small incision made earlier and touches it gently to the hardened cataract lens.
4. A small portion of the iris is slit to facilitate removal of the lens. This is rarely done with forceps, as it once was, but with a freeeze probe that quick-freezes to the lens the way your finger sometimes sticks to a cold metal ice-cube tray. Then the freeze probe, the lens stuck firmly to it, is withdrawn through the slit in the iris.	4. The ultrasound probe is activated, quickly vibrating the cataract first into minute particles, then into a liquid. At the same time, fluid is released through the ultrasound instrument to wash through the eye. Then the cataract, now in liquid state, and the fluid wash are sucked out of the eye through the hollow ultrasound probe. The cataract has been removed, and the probe is withdrawn.
5. The 3/4″ incision is sewn shut with eight or more stitches, which will be removed later, perhaps longer.	5. The 1/16″ incision is sewn shut with a single stitch that need never be removed since it will dissolve by itself.
6. Operating time: generally 30 minutes to an hour.	6. Operating time: generally less than 10 to 12 minutes.

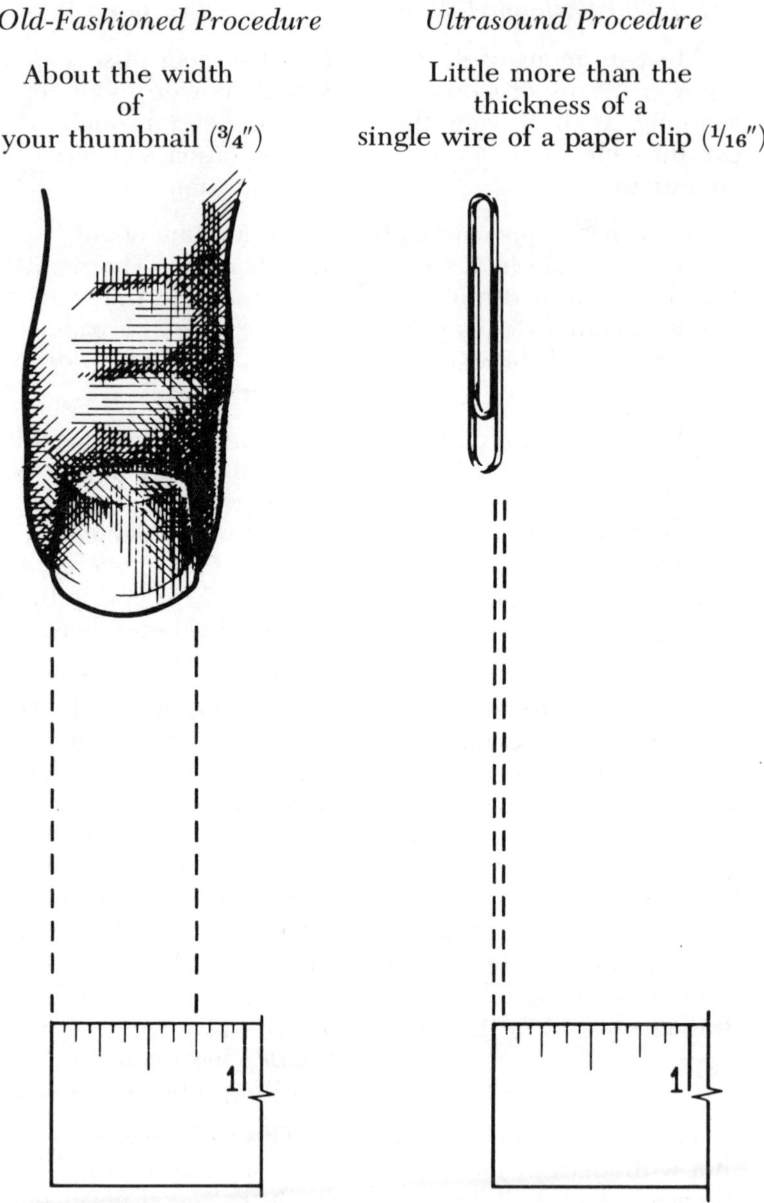

Figure 1. *How the two procedures compare.*

But as you can see, there are considerable differences between them. One important difference has to do with trauma.

Trauma, in simple terms, means injury. And with injury comes pain. The larger the incision, the more disturbed the affected area—in this case, the eye—becomes, the greater the trauma. And the eye is a very sensitive area.

One of the great benefits of ultrasound cataract surgery is that there is very little disturbance to the eye. The tiny incision, the use of high-powered microsurgery, the fine little single stitch, these add up to a minimal amount of trauma, less chance of possible damage to the cornea, and a far speedier return of the eye to normal functioning.

Now, when anyone considers an operation, any kind of operation, there most naturally comes to mind a worry about bleeding. But eye surgery for cataracts is totally unlike abdominal surgery or heart surgery or operative procedures on other organs of the body.

The blood vessels of the eye are so tiny that there is ordinarily no bleeding at all.

Remember, too, that in ultrasound cataract surgery, that little probe and all the other instruments are miniaturized. They are so small that only a high-powered microscope makes their use possible.

There is a good-sized console supplying the power during the operation that dwarfs the pencil-like probe I hold in my gloved hand. The console is computerized to measure out precisely and instantaneously the power needed to make the probe's tip vibrate at the necessary high frequency, and the pressure needed to irrigate the eye with fluid and then suck out the liquefied cataract.

With a single foot pedal, I am able to issue orders to the computer to release fluid into the eye, time the amount of ultrasound needed for that particular cataract, and draw the emulsified lens out of the eye.

Buzz-buzz-buzz, and it is all over.

If I appear to be biased in favor of ultrasound, I am. For the reasons I have already mentioned in some detail. And also from my experience with patients who have had one cataract removed the old-fashioned way and the other removed by ultrasound.

Nevertheless, I want to assure all of you who are experiencing anxiety about undergoing cataract surgery that both procedures produce good results in the long run. I have no desire to shake your confidence in the eye surgeon you have chosen to do the operation, no matter what procedure he follows.

But I must make an exception in the case of a congenital cataract, the kind some children are born with. The cause of such cataracts is obscure. It is thought that it may be associated with the mother's having rubella (German measles) during pregnancy. Then, too, there is a common triad, still not completely understood, in which a child is born with heart disease, ear defects, and congenital cataracts.

The point I wish to make is that such a cataract can be very dense, but the ligaments that I referred to earlier are very strong in a child. They are attached firmly to several structures in the eye, and they are not easily loosened. This is why traditional surgery should not be done on congenital cataracts.

The medication, the enzyme, used in such surgery to loosen those ligaments does not loosen the other attachments in the eye that tie the lens to other parts of the eye, such as the vitreous, the jellylike substance behind the lens.

Therefore, when the lens is pulled out, as it is in traditional cataract surgery, other structures may be pulled out as well. The whole thing is like a tug of war. The doctor pulls, the structures resist, and the eye could be lost.

This is not the case with ultrasound surgery, which, as I mentioned, is based on the technique called phacoemulsification. Remember, the word "phaco" in Greek means "lens," and the word "emulsification" means "reducing a solid to a liquid." By reducing that solid cataract lens to a liquid, those tough ligaments in a child's eye remain undisturbed. There is no tug of war.

Would you believe, or even suspect, that a 10-month-old child could undergo cataract surgery successfully?

Well, let me tell you about a little girl named

Gina, the daughter of Navy Cmdr. and Mrs. Ernie Tedeschi. Her cataracts were present at birth but went undetected until she was almost 10 months old.

At that time, her parents noticed a cloudiness in her right eye. They watched it, and it quickly worsened. So they rushed her to a clinic where she was given 12 hours of exhaustive testing and was diagnosed as having cataracts in both eyes.

For all intents and purposes, the child was legally blind.

"It was an incredible shock," her father told me when he decided to bring her to my office at Germantown Hospital. "She had been a superhealthy baby."

They had been referred to me by another doctor after having been told by the clinic doctors that while surgery was imperative, Gina would never have better than 20/70 vision, which means that she would see at 20 feet what normal people could see at 70 feet. This did not satisfy her parents.

Moreover, there was the possibility that cataracts in such a young child could recur, in the sense that their complete removal by traditional techniques might require two, three, or even four operations.

I was confident that I could take care of the cataracts in a single operation and with little or no discomfort to the child, using ultrasound surgery. But I told her parents frankly that it was impossible to calculate for certain if her vision would ultimately be perfect. Much depended on how healthy her eyes were, aside from the cataracts that had caused her blindness.

Everything went beautifully. I felt especially good because little Gina was my youngest patient at that time. When the effects of the operation wore off, and her eyes began to heal, I fitted her with soft contact lenses, perfect in her case. As she matures, that lens prescription will be changed, and she will indeed have 20/20 vision.

This brings up another aspect of cataract surgery—the healing process, and how it differs in the two procedures, and how it affects you no matter what your age.

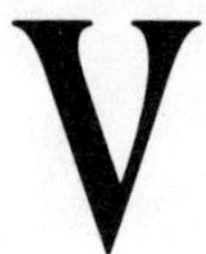

How Your Sight Will Return

Now that your cataract has been removed, it is gone forever. It will never grow back again.

I take pains to make this clear to all my patients before surgery because, even if they don't ask the question directly, I know from experience that it is on their minds. It is important for their peace of mind to understand that once that cataract is removed—by the ultrasound procedure that I prefer or by the old-fashioned procedure—it is gone for good.

If you were my patient, I would tell you, "That clouded, hardened lens will never trouble you again."

All right, the operation is over. And now you are wondering, "How does healing take place?

What happens after the operation? How long will it take for me to regain my sight?"

These are some of the questions I will discuss in this chapter. And I can tell you right now that if you enjoyed perfect vision before you had a cataract, you will very likely regain equally good vision after that cataract is removed.

But there is a decided difference in the way recovery takes place after the ultrasound procedure and the traditional, old-fashioned procedure.

Let us return to our side-by-side comparison of the two procedures, but this time in terms of the recovery process. Picture yourself as the patient. The operation is over. It is successful. Your cataract is gone. You are on your way now to the recovery room. Here is what happens next.

The Old-Fashioned Way	*The Ultrasound Way*
1) You sleep off the tranquilizer and anesthetic, which might require several hours to wear off because of the larger incision made.	1) You sleep off the tranquilizer and anesthetic, which usually wears off quickly as the eye was less disturbed in surgery.
2) Your operated eye is always covered with a patch to prevent your accidentally poking a finger into the eye.	2) Your operated eye is not covered. There is no need for it since only one stitch closed the small incision.
3) You return to your hospital room and are put to bed. You will be hospitalized for from 5 to 10 days, although you may be permitted out of bed within a day or two.	3) You can go home two hours after the operation. If you have other medical problems or are elderly, you might be encouraged to stay overnight.

The Old-Fashioned Way	*The Ultrasound Way*
4) You may be fitted with temporary cataract glasses after your hospital stay but restricted in your activities to avoid wound problems.	4) You will be fitted with temporary cataract glasses, able to perform near-normal activities, immediately after surgery. No restrictions are necessary.
5) The sutures (stitches) are checked daily during your hospitalization, then weekly for from 6 to 15 weeks.	5) The single suture is checked only twice: two days after the operation, and again at the end of a week.
6) After a healing period of eight weeks or more, prescription lenses can be prescribed to restore the sight you had before you had the cataract.	6) Prescription lenses can be prescribed as a rule within two to three weeks after surgery to restore your sight to what it was before you had the cataract.

In brief, then, those are the essential differences between the two procedures following cataract surgery. Rest assured that either procedure can successfully restore your sight.

With the ultrasound procedure, however, that the eye is less disturbed makes unnecessary the kinds of restrictions imposed by the old-fashioned operation. You are able to get around more quickly, avoid a long hospital stay, and not worry about coughing, lifting, or otherwise disturbing the operated eye.

Let me give you an example of a typical patient who underwent ultrasound surgery. Her name is Natalie Finley. She is quite knowledgeable about eye problems inasmuch as she is employed as an assistant to an optometrist.

"I want to get rid of this cataract because it's interfering with my work," she told me. "But I don't want to go through the long wait of conventional surgery. A friend of mine went through it, and even after six weeks, she still couldn't see clearly."

After examining her eyes carefully, I assured her that there would be no complications and that she would waste little time getting back to her job.

On the day of her operation, she went first to her office, turned on the lights, adjusted the heat, and set up the day's appointments for the optometrist she worked for. Then, instead of taking her usual lunch break, she came to Germantown Hospital.

Two hours later, she was able to return to her office, type a letter, and then take the rest of the day off. She was in excellent health, and it was not necessary for me to give her more than minimal sedation prior to surgery; of course, it wore off fast.

"I was completely awake during the operation," she told me later, "but didn't feel a thing. In fact, when it was all over, I really felt so good I could have played golf if the weather had been good and if I hadn't had to go back to my office to take care of some unfinished business."

When I send patients like Mrs. Finley home after surgery, I give them eyedrops combining an antibiotic with a harmless steroid to make the eye more comfortable and promote healing. I also give them an irrigating solution, an eyewash, to cleanse their eyelids if necessary. These are all painless procedures.

Now I don't like to talk about pain because it inspires fear in cataract patients, but I believe I owe it to my readers to discuss it in this book.

As far as cataract surgery goes, I want to say right here that both procedures are absolutely painless. There may be some differences after the operation due to the fact that conventional surgery is more disturbing to the eye, since it requires a much larger incision, more stitches, and a different technique in removing the clouded lens. Because of this, there is more trauma, as I mentioned in the previous chapter.

Nevertheless, pain is almost nonexistent in cataract surgery. For one thing, experiencing pain is something very personal, depending on a particular patient's sensitivity. What is merely a slight irritation to one person could be a more than mild annoyance to another.

In other words, pain is often relative.

But there is more to it than that. Say, for example, that you are in the kitchen stuffing a turkey and you prick your finger with a skewer. It hurts. In a few moments, however, the hurt is gone, and the bleeding has stopped.

So you proceed to pick up a sharp knife and cut up those vegetables to go with your dinner. In the process, your knife slips, and you slice your finger instead of the carrots. Now it will take several hours before your finger stops throbbing, and you will probably have to wear a bandage for a few days. The pain, too, will be more severe from the knife slice than from the prick of the skewer.

In a way, this is the difference between ultrasound and traditional operations. Because ultrasound requires only a tiny opening and a single stitch, the recovery process is very much shortened, as is the discomfort.

Following surgery, with either operation, you will feel no pain but some brief discomfort, as though there is something in your eye. This is controlled easily by mild medication, even aspirin. Naturally, with the larger incision, you may experience more discomfort.

In any case, it is not a painful condition, merely an annoyance. This is important for anyone contemplating cataract surgery to understand.

You should understand, too, that all cataract surgery has improved tremendously just over the last decade. For example, it is not unlikely that you have heard somewhere that following the operation, you must lie still in bed with your head between sandbags to prevent moving your head.

That was true at one time, but is not true today. Even with the old-fashioned operation, you can be up and around within a reasonable time. But even today you will have to restrict your activities with the traditional operation.

You will have to be careful about lifting things, bending over, touching your hand to your eye, or even pressing yourself on the toilet to move your bowels. These precautions are necessary to prevent the eye sutures from popping out due to undue strain.

This does not mean that I am going to tell you to jog home after ultrasound surgery and go bowling that evening. But you will be able to get back to being your normal self much faster, tie your shoelaces without worrying about bending over, go about most of your business, and—within a few days—jog again, play tennis, or drive again.

I am often asked by my patients, "Is it all right for me to smoke or drink?"

I tell them, yes, of course, you can smoke if you like, and you can have a drink if you like. No problem.

Some of my female patients are concerned about going to the beauty parlor to have their hair done. The reason is that with the traditional operation it may be unwise to bend your head backward or forward. Ultrasound surgery eliminates such problems. If you are a woman and concerned about your appearance, you need not wait weeks or months to visit your favorite beauty parlor; you can have your hair done the next day.

I am also asked by many patients, "Do I have to follow any kind of special diet after the operation?"

My answer is, "No, absolutely not. Eat whatever you like. Your operation has nothing to do with your appetite or your digestive processes!"

Nor do you have to wear dark glasses after the operation even though colors may appear more vivid. This may be because the human lens filters out wavelengths of light that are not filtered out by its replacement, whether it is a cataract glass, a contact lens, or an artificial lens implant.

A common misconception about cataract surgery concerns the ability to see immediately or shortly after the operation. I want to talk about this right here.

When your eye is operated on, there is some swelling. This swelling goes away gradually. When you start out with a cataract that is so dense it only permits you to see light, you will see a whole lot more within hours after the anesthetic wears off in the ultrasound procedure.

You should be able to see forms, a hand in front of you, count fingers, or even read large letters. That is a tremendous improvement over a cataract so dense that it could admit only light and nothing more!

Naturally, if your cataract was not so dense, your vision would be much better following surgery. That veil that disorted your vision would be gone. Even temporary glasses would give you seeing ability that you have not enjoyed in years. And your vision will continually improve as the eye heals.

With traditional surgery, of course, the healing process takes longer. But this does not mean that you will not get back good vision. It only means that it will take longer.

It is wrong to believe that you cannot see without prescription glasses, contact lenses, or even intraocular lens implants. You can see after the operation, but not as clearly as you would with the human lens, which focused the visual images on your retina. Clarity comes after you are fitted with temporary lenses, which give usable vision almost immediately following ultrasound surgery or within a week or so following traditional surgery. An artificial lens implant can restore clarity much sooner, but more about that later.

Keep in mind that it takes a while for vision to build up. And there are some cases in which swelling of eye tissue retards the return of good sight at the beginning of the recovery period, perhaps for several days, but this is rare. In 9 out of 10 cases, you start to see better almost at once.

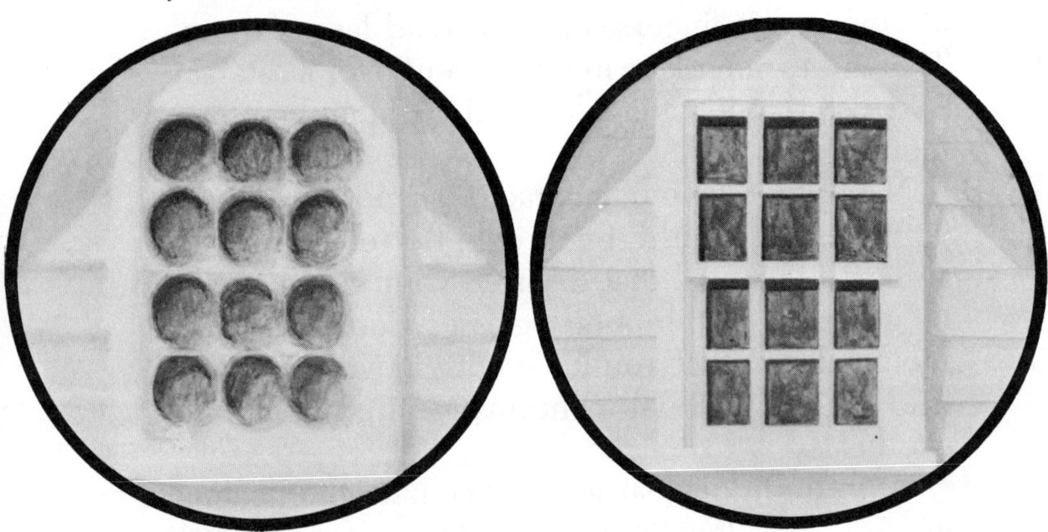

Without a Corrective Lens *With a Corrective Lens*

Figure 2. *How you will see after cataract surgery.* The corrective lens could be a permanent lens implant, a contact lens, or cataract glasses. In some situations, no corrective lens is needed, as explained in Chapter VII.

I think it is comforting to hear about other cataract victims who have undergone surgery, and so I am going to dip into my patient file again to tell you about Richard Dempsey, who consulted me for a second cataract operation.

He had undergone his first cataract operation by the old-fashioned procedure and told me, "It worked out fine, but it took me three months to recover. I don't want to go through that again."

It was a challenge to me. There was no doubt that the cataract in his other eye needed to be extracted and that Mr. Dempsey was impatient that his full sight be restored as quickly as possible.

The operation took but minutes, and I was able to say to him, "Your cataract's gone, Richard. Did you feel anything?"

"I heard a buzz while you were operating," he said, "but I didn't feel anything at all."

He was a bit groggy from the tranquilizer, so I had him sit around until the drug had worn off. Before two hours had passed, following the operation, I examined his eye and said, "Everything looks fine. You can go home now and do anything you did before the operation. Meanwhile, use your other eye. When I see you again, we'll fit you with a contact lens to bring your vision back to normal."

It was a normal procedure and is typical of 95 percent of the cases that come to my attention. I think this also might be the time to mention that the ultrasound procedure has received full approval and support from the American Academy of Ophthalmology, the federal government's Department of Health, Education and Welfare, and is eligible under Medicare.

I think it is also appropriate to mention here that perhaps 1 out of 20 cataract patients—more after traditional surgery—may experience what is known medically as ptosis. In laymen's language, this means simply that the eyelid of the operated eye droops.

It is nothing to be alarmed about should it occur. It is generally due to a weakness in the eyelid muscle, which has been exacerbated by the incision and sutures, inflaming the inner lining of the eyelid. Naturally, the greater the incision and the more stitches, the greater the inflammation, which is why it is more prevalent with traditional surgery.

But, in any case, it is almost always a temporary condition that will disappear in time. It has nothing to do with the restoration of your sight and is nothing to be concerned about.

To reassure you further, let me advise you that the ultrasound procedure has been employed successfully on more than half a million cataract patients, so you can choose it with confidence if you require cataract surgery.

This leaves only the problem of how to replace the removed cataract lens. Should you choose cataract glasses, contact lenses, or decide, preferably before the operation, to have intraocular lens implants?

The lens implant offers a great many advantages, and for some people it could be an absolute necessity, as I will point out in the next chapter. But even contact lenses and cataract glasses can restore vision effectively. The choice depends on both your personal preference and your particular needs.

VI

Seeing Again With a Substitute Lens

That cataract you had taken out was a lens, a clouded lens that prevented you from seeing clearly. Without it, you have what is known medically as "aphakic vision," which means nothing more than lens-less vision. Your eye does not have the power of accommodation it needs for it to produce the kind of clear focus you once enjoyed.

You need a new clear lens to replace that clouded one.

That, in a nutshell, is the essence of cataract surgery. It is a simple exchange. You have the bad lens taken out and get back a new one in return.

You can wear that new lens just as you would ordinary eyeglasses by ordering cataract spectacles. Or you could wear a contact lens, hard or soft, and dispense with the need for spectacles. Or you could have a new lens implanted permanently in place of the old clouded one and dispense with the need for either contacts or spectacles for general viewing.

But whatever your decision, it should be made prior to the operation. You should have a clear understanding of the differences among these three choices before consenting to surgery, for this is a most important decision and one that must be made on an individual basis. What is best for one person is not necessarily best for another.

Your goal is to get back the good vision you had before you had a cataract and to do so with the least possible discomfort to yourself.

What this means is that psychological as well as physiological factors must be taken into consideration.

Some cataract patients, for example, may not have all three options to choose from. For one reason or another—and we will explore some of these reasons in this chapter—they may be restricted to two, or even only one, of these choices.

It is part of your doctor's job to make it crystal clear to you beforehand what choices are available to you and why he believes one should be chosen above the others.

If I seem to belabor this point, please forgive me. But from my experience, and the previous experiences of many of my patients, I have learned that all too many eye doctors do not take the time to discuss this matter thoroughly enough. A great many, for example, do not even mention

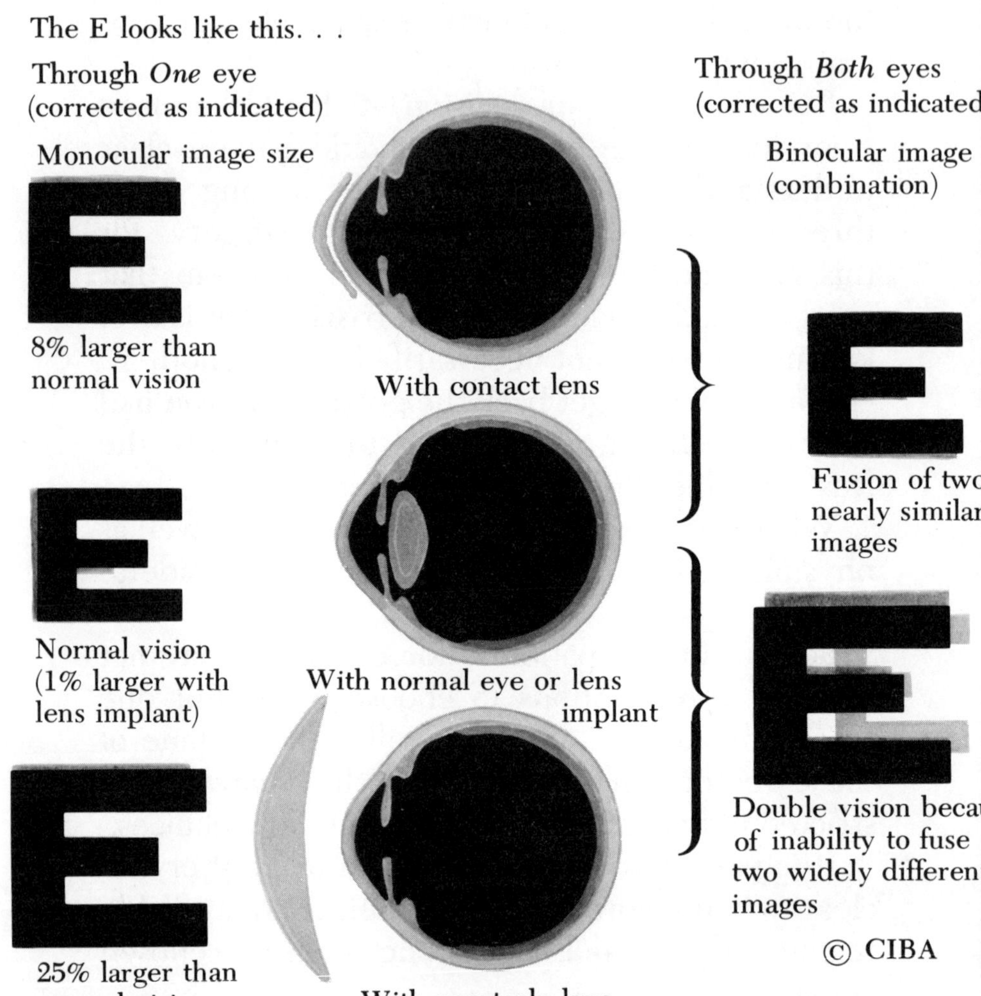

Figure 3. *How you will see through different corrective lenses—for one or both eyes, after cataract surgery.*

the possibility of an artificial lens implant, which would be ideal for many patients, simply because they are not practiced in this procedure. Yet it might be the very best choice for you. I will have more to say about this in a later chapter.

But now let us consider the three choices, one at a time, so that you will know the advantages and limitations of each. For while all are effective in restoring good vision, there is only one that is best for you.

If you are to make a truly informed decision, you should know how spectacles, contacts, and implants differ in their roles as substitute lenses.

Cataract Spectacles

The eyeglasses available today for cataract patients are not what used to be known as "Coke-bottle" glasses—because their thick bulging lenses resembled the bottom of a Coca-Cola bottle.

The lenses in modern cataract glasses are lighter in weight and frequently made of plastic, which is ground to prescription specifications. Nevertheless, they are heavier than ordinary spectacles and must be worn at a precise distance from the eye. You can not push them up and down over your nose as you can ordinary eyeglasses if you want good corrected vision.

Here is why:

That clouded cataract lens you had taken out was inside your eye. But the replacement lenses in cataract spectacles, just as lenses in any spectacles, are worn outside your eyes, in front of them.

This increases the distance between them and the retina, that movie screen in your eye on which everything you see is projected.

Because of this increased distance, the image projected on the retina will be larger, almost one and one-half times larger, than normal. As a result, everything you see will appear larger than lifesize.

This will take some getting used to. Things will seem closer to you than they really are. Everything from the cup and saucer on your breakfast table to the stoplight across the street.

What this means to you, if you wear cataract spectacles, is that you have to learn to rejudge distances.

It is really not that difficult. Many people get along very well with cataract spectacles, but this aspect should be taken into consideration with this choice.

There is something else you should know about cataract spectacles. In the very first chapter of this book, I mentioned that these glasses restrict side vision by two-thirds. Another name for side vision is peripheral vision.

You can see clearly, but only what is directly in front of you. You cannot see what is going on to either side. This is why some wearers of cataract glasses say it is like looking through the hole in a doughnut.

If you want to see what is going on outside that hole, you cannot simply shift your eyeball left or right. You have to turn your head left or right.

But this, too, is something you can get used to. It has nothing to do with your ability to see clearly, but to do so, you must look straight ahead.

These are some of the disadvantages of cataract spectacles. Let me assure you, however, that these are not by any means insurmountable obstacles. A bit of patience can help you overcome these shortcomings.

To use cataract spectacles successfully, however, you must have had both eyes operated on. There is no way you can use both eyes together with cataract glasses after one operation.

Why? Because you will be seeing a much larger image through the cataract glass with the operated eye from which the clouded lens was removed. Your brain cannot fuse together this larger image with the normal-sized image you see through your unoperated eye.

You will see double, a condition known as "diplopia."

So if you have a cataract only in one eye, and the other eye is normal, you cannot elect cataract spectacles. You must choose either a contact lens or an artificial lens implant for the operated eye.

This is something that should be very carefully explained to anyone contemplating a cataract procedure, whether by the old-fashioned method or by the ultrasound technique.

Unfortunately, too many eye doctors neglect to make this clear to their patients. This is one reason why I decided to write this book and presumably why you decided to read it: to answer the kinds of questions cataract patients fail to ask and doctors do not explain sufficiently.

For some people, cataract spectacles are the best choice, perhaps even the only one. Remember my mentioning the gentleman named Jesse Yoder in the second chapter of this book? He had already had one cataract removed by the old-fashioned procedure before he came to me for extraction of a cataract in his other eye.

He was having difficulty using a contact lens in the first eye, and he would have to keep using it if I gave him a lens implant in the second eye. So his best choice was cataract spectacles, which he found perfect for both eyes.

You might also want to turn back to the third chapter in which I talked about another patient, Joseph B. Van Sciver, Jr. Since he could not see at all through one eye, he was able to wear cataract spectacles after I removed the cataract from the other eye.

Since he was only seeing through one eye after surgery, there was no problem of double vision with cataract glasses. They gave him perfect 20/20 vision on that one operated eye, and he said that was sufficient for him.

Before leaving the subject of cataract spectacles, I want to distinguish between using them permanently and using them for a very short time. Immediately after the ultrasound procedure, if you do not choose to have a lens implant, I might fit you with temporary glasses to help you see better more quickly.

With your cataract gone, that veil that disturbed your vision is gone. And with temporary glasses you might be able to see better, read the eye chart better, within a matter of hours. If you had an implant, you could expect to regain normal vision much more quickly.

For example, if you saw well up close before you had the cataract, you would very likely tell me, "Hey, doc, you know, I can read again!" Or if you saw distances well before you had a cataract, you would say, "Hey, doc, I can look out my window and see the signs on the street again!"

But with or without the implant, I might recommend temporary glasses. But they would only be just that, temporary, to bridge the gap between removal of your cataract and full restoration of your vision.

Contact Lenses

For many people, contact lenses are a better choice than cataract spectacles. Since they rest directly on the eye, they are much closer to the retina than are cataract glasses. Therefore, they give only a slightly enlarged image and good side vision.

With contact lenses, you can expect little or no difficulty rejudging distances, and you do not experience the effect of peering through the hole of a doughnut.

The trouble, if any, with contact lenses is that they are troublesome to some people. You do have to pop them in and out of your eye. And you may be the sort who dislikes the business of inserting anything, even very thin contact lenses, into your eye. Psychologically, you may have difficulty doing this.

There are also purely physical barriers to wearing contacts. You may have a shaky hand, or perhaps you are bothered by arthritis in your fingers; managing contacts could then be more than you could handle.

And here is something else that few doctors bother to tell their patients. While they will inform you that your operated eye will see fine again with a contact lens, they will neglect to inform you that if your other eye is bad you will be unable to look at your mirror to fit that contact lens in the operated eye.

Think about that for a moment. The only eye with vision is the operated one. That is the eye in which you have to insert the contact lens. But you are unable to see through the other eye to do it. Someone has to do it for you.

A better solution might be to use cataract glasses, which you can do because you have the use of only one eye. When the cataract is removed from your other eye, then you can discard the cataract glasses and switch over to contact lenses because then you will be able to see what you are doing.

This has nothing to do with the quality of vision that a contact lens will give you but only with the business of popping that contact in and out of your eye.

Now let us talk a bit about the situation in which you have one eye that sees well and another that has a cataract. You have the cataract removed and, for one reason or another, have decided against having that clouded lens replaced by an artificial lens implant.

You cannot wear cataract glasses because you would then have double vision, as I explained earlier. You can, however, wear a contact lens in the operated eye, and because the contact does not enlarge images the way cataract spectacles do, your brain can fuse the two images so that you will see clearly again.

That is an important distinction between spectacles and contacts.

With these caveats in mind. I would say that middle-aged cataract patients ordinarily should do well with contact lenses.

If you were my patient, I would want to discuss your feelings about contact lenses before surgery. If you were elderly, I would do all I could to persuade you to have a lens implant instead, to avoid a situation in which you would need a contact lens to see but could not wear it.

And even if you were not elderly, I would like the option of putting in an implant when I remove your cataract if I saw that it would be proper and easy to do so. Naturally, if there was any question that it would be difficult, I would never do it. But I would want you to sign a consent form to allow me that option, to make that decision in your own best interests as your doctor.

Let me dip into my patient file to illustrate my point. A gentleman named John Keene consulted me about a cataract and had every expectation of replacing the clouded lens with a permanent intraocular artificial lens implant.

However, on careful examination of his eye before the operation, I saw that the implant would not be practical for him. He was one of those few persons—and they are very few—who had too little natural space in the eye between the cornea and the iris to properly accommodate even the miniscule artificial lens.

But he could manage a contact lens very well, and that was the option I recommended. I prescribed a soft contact because it was water absorbent and would be easier for him to adapt to. At the same time, I advised him that soft contacts needed more caring for—they have to be kept wetted down, for example—but he did not regard this as a particular problem.

Similarly, I fitted another patient, William Reifsnyder, with contact lenses, also of the soft kind, not because he could not have lens implants, but because he preferred contacts.

I commenced the ultrasound procedure at 11:45 in the morning. He was out of the operating room and fully awake at 12:20 that same day and back home two hours later. He wears soft contacts, likes them, has 20/20 vision, and leads a normal life.

Please understand that you cannot be fitted with contact lenses immediately after the operation. You will be fitted much sooner after the ultrasound procedure than after the old-fashioned operation. And you will have sight, as I explained in the previous chapter. But you may have to put up with temporary cataract spectacles for a brief period, usually no longer than two or three weeks, before contacts can be prescribed.

Now I would like to say something about what are called "full-time contacts," which never have to be removed. These do exist, but I do not often recommend them.

When you leave something in your eye, pressing against the cornea, for a long period of time, that cornea does not get all the oxygen it needs to thrive. The cornea is living tissue, and living tissue requires oxygen. Without it, new blood vessels can grow in progressively at the edge of the cornea. That will eventually affect your vision.

For this reason, I am reluctant to recommend the use of full-time contacts. They might be fine in special situations, as for the very elderly patient. But they are unthinkable for younger patients.

Permanent Lens Implants

The greatest advance in cataract surgery, aside from the ultrasound procedure, is the development of the artificial lens implant. Professionally, it is known as an intraocular lens because it is slipped directly into the eye and becomes a part of the eye.

With it, you might have to wait no more than 24 hours to experience normal vision. You can look forward to seeing objects in their normal size (actually, 1 percent larger, but this is a negligible difference). You will enjoy normal depth perception, perfect side vision, and no distortion.

Moreover, if you had a cataract only in one eye, that eye, with an implant, will team up just about perfectly with the other eye so that you can enjoy good vision once again with both eyes. All this without cataract glasses or contact lenses. And that implanted lens works 24 hours a day for all time, correcting your sight permanently.

I have found that that does wonders for people's morale as well as for their vision.

A distinguished professional publication, *The Medical Letter*, published by doctors for doctors, put it this way:

> The advantages of intraocular lenses over contact lenses and aphakic spectacles for patients who have had cataracts removed are full visual fields, little magnification of images, 24-hour use, good uncorrected vision, better depth perception, binocular vision when only one cataract has been removed, and absence of discomfort or inconvenience caused by environmental dust and chemicals.

They go on to cite a study that showed "100 consecutive implantations produced excellent visual results" and that "80 percent of the patients had visual acuity of 20/20 or 20/25."

This agrees with my own experience after implanting more than 1,000 artificial lenses.

I want to tell you about a very charming lady named Mrs. Kathryn Darlington. Her son brought her to see me at Germantown Hospital after she had told him, "I saw a story about this doctor's way of operating on cataracts in a Philadelphia newspaper, and I clipped it and filed it. I didn't really want to have an operation. But now that my eyes are so bad I'm just falling around, I think I ought to talk to him."

This is very typical of people with cataracts. They are so fearful of the procedure that they keep putting it off until they reach the point that Mrs. Darlington had reached, where her vision had deteriorated so far that she was "stumbling around," as she expressed it.

I spent a good deal of time speaking to her and her son, explaining the procedure, examining her eyes, and reassuring both of them, detailing just what would be done, how it would be done, and why I thought she was a good candidate for a lens implant. I even showed her the apparatus used in ultrasound surgery. She was awed by the size of the equipment needed to operate on an eye and said, "Oh, my goodness, it's almost as big as the room!"

This helped greatly in lessening her fear. She told me later, "It only took that one visit to convince me. That's why I made the appointment for the operation right then and there."

I did the usual two-step procedure: first the ultrasound procedure to remove the cataract and then the insertion of the lens implant. It was all done under local anesthesia, so that she recovered very quickly and could judge the results almost immediately. Even without glasses, she found herself able to see.

"Right after I got home," she told me, "I was able to stoop over and feed my dogs and cats. I could look in the mirror and see my own eye, which I hadn't been able to do for some time."

The implant has made a lot of difference in her life. It has presented no problems. Quite the contrary. It has enabled her to once again become self-sufficient. That is her style. "I'm used to looking out for myself," she told me. And that is why I deemed it important to explain to her in some detail exactly what the procedure entailed.

The plastic lens I use for an implant is very small, about an eighth of an inch wide, and is made of polymethylmethacrilate of superior clinical quality.

When I place the implant in your eye, I hold it in my right hand while holding the cornea open just a little bit with my left hand and slide the implant into place right there in the part of the capsule I talked about earlier. It is held fast with tiny loops made of a substance called Prolene, a derivative of nylon that does not degenerate.

That is all there is to it.

Of course, it is all done under the operating microscope, the only way to do such a delicate procedure. Surgeons who do not use a microscope must use a larger, less sophisticated lens, and that is not something I would recommend.

The entire procedure can be compared to removing a ball from a cellophane wrapper. Imagine yourself opening up only enough of the cellophane to take out the ball, leaving the rest of the cellophane wrapper intact, into which you can drop a new ball to replace the defective one.

Call the cellophane the membrane, call the defective old ball the cataract, call the new ball the artificial lens implant, and you will have a pretty good idea of how it is all done.

But with old-fashioned cataract surgery, the entire membrane, that whole piece of cellophane, is removed. There is nothing left to hold the implant. It has to be hung with clips on the iris and the jellylike part of the eye called the vitreous, and this kind of support can give way in time.

You might be interested to know that the intraocular lens resulted from a fluke, a chance observation made by a prominent British ophthalmologist, Dr. Harold Ridley, during World War II.

Dr. Ridley noticed that British pilots who had been in combat often had bits of plastic material in their eyes. This plastic material came from the canopies of their Spitfire airplanes.

Astonishingly, however, Dr. Ridley discovered that these bits of plastic did not bother the fighter pilots' eyes. They just stayed inert, with no complications occurring even over a period of 20 years.

Thus did Dr. Ridley initiate the first experiments with artificial plastic lens implants.

We have come a long way since then. Implant procedures are now greatly refined, perfected, particularly in combination with ultrasound removal of cataracts, to the point at which an ophthalmologist need no longer say to a patient, merely, "You have a cataract, it must be removed."

He can indeed say, "Your eye needs a new lens. We can insert one for you."

But there is a considerable difference between lens implant procedures, just as there is between cataract extraction procedures. I have already made some references to these differences. I want to make one more.

In the old-fashioned, or conventional, cataract operation, the lens implant procedure depends on clips, sutures, and various ways of attaching the intraocular lens.

Now please think about that for a moment.

If there are so many different ways to attach the artificial lens to the iris, it follows that there is no one good way.

With the ultrasound procedure, there is only one way to put an artificial plastic lens in place. Only one good way.

That makes a big difference.

With the ultrasound procedure, the chances of a lens implant coming loose are almost miniscule. In the more than a thousand implants I have done, I have had a lens come loose only five times, and then it was simply a matter of slipping that lens back into place and sealing it there for good. No problem.

Oh, yes, I will tell you after lens implantation to

take care not to rub your eye and, depending on your particular situation, may advise you against undertaking strenuous work.

But I will not stop you from watching television and reading or make you wear an eye shield or keep you hospitalized for days or even weeks.

No operative procedure is a bed of roses, but the possibility of complications with ultrasound surgery and lens implantation is extremely low, possibly 3 percent.

I will ask you to come back to see me within a few days after the procedure to check how your new lens is doing. In almost 100 percent of my patients, that checkup reveals that the new lens is firmly anchored, and all restrictions are lifted.

You can now resume your customary life style and do anything you want.

Some people tend to compare a lens implant with an organ transplant such as an artificial kidney. Well, the two are quite different.

An artificial lens in no way can be compared to an artificial kidney or a heart transplant. It does not need a blood supply to keep it working. In fact, it has to remain clear. And there are no blood vessels circulating around it. These would bring in antibodies, as in the case of transplants, which contribute to the problem of rejection.

There is no possibility that a lens implant can be rejected. Be assured of this. It is not implanted in tissue. It is isolated in fluid. That is the difference.

And please do not confuse an intraocular implant with a silicone implant. They are totally different, too. And this difference exists no matter how it is implanted, whether by the old-fashioned procedure or in conjunction with the ultrasound procedure.

Despite the many advantages of an implant to replace the cataract lens, some patients cannot—and should not—elect them.

If you have a condition known as chronic iritis, such as it is believed that Elvis Presley experienced, I would be reluctant to give you an implant. If you had one or two bouts of iritis that cleared up easily, I might do it. But if the iritis cannot be cleared up, I would try to avoid any kind of cataract surgery at all. This applies doubly to conventional surgery, which entails much suturing of the iris that is already inflamed.

If you have what is known medically as shallow anterior chambers, meaning that the space between the cornea and the iris is smaller than usual, as in the case of Mr. John Keene, mentioned earlier, I would have to be sure that the space was sufficient to accommodate a new lens. Using conventional surgery, I would not be able to do it. With ultrasound surgery, I might be able to in most cases.

If you suffer from what is called corneal endothelial dystrophy—damaged cells inside the cornea—it might prohibit lens implantation or even basic cataract surgery. My decision would depend on how severe or how mild the damage is. If it is mild, I would not expect to have any problem. But first I would carefully examine your eyes to ascertain just how extensive the damage is.

If you have a detached retina, I would be very cautious about recommending a lens implant.

If you have glaucoma, but it is controlled, you can have an implant.

If you have diabetes with complications, you still might have an implant, but the diabetes complications will be more difficult to treat. That does not mean that such problems cannot be treated, only that they will present more difficulty to the doctor.

There are situations in which an implant is simply unnecessary because your eye is so structured that you will be able to see perfectly well without it and without cataract glasses or contact lenses. I will talk about this in the next chapter.

You may read that the FDA (Food and Drug Administration) is checking into the safety of intraocular lenses. This is true, but it has to do with the medical devices legislation authorized by Congress. It is concerned only with the artificial lens itself and the manufacturer of that lens.

I am one of the ophthalmologists involved in this particular study. It is the same sort of study that determines the effectiveness and safety of other medical devices, such as cardiac pacemakers, intrauterine devices, and even contact lenses. It is simply a check on the manufacturers of lens implants and has nothing to do with the safety of lens implantation.

It is only a means of protecting you against the use of substandard medical devices of any kind. That is all. So be assured that if you elect a permanent lens implant, you have nothing to worry about. A good eye surgeon knows which lens is safe, and that is the only one he will use.

VII

Some Very Special Cataracts

Aside from cataracts that develop over the years and the congenital kind with which some children are born, there is a cataract that results from trauma—that is, injury to the eye. It might arise with what seems to be startling suddenness or mature insidiously.

This was the experience of Mrs. Phyllis Baker, the victim of an automobile accident. She had traumatic cataracts, and the one in her right eye was progressing rapidly. But the eye doctor whom she consulted advised her to wait, that it might take years before the cataracts could be removed because they were not yet "ripe."

She did not have to wait very long before she lost all vision in that right eye. A business woman engaged in custom crafts work—ceramics and handmade crocheted and knitted goods—she found herself unable to keep on with her work without the use of both eyes.

She had heard about my work with ultrasound and lens implants and telephoned me for an appointment. "I have to get my sight back," she said, "but I don't want to wear special eyeglasses or contact lenses. Can you help me if I fly in to Philadelphia to see you?"

Naturally, I could not give her a responsible answer on the telephone no matter how much information she gave me. All I could say was that very possibly I could try to relieve some of her anxiety, and tell her that she had to let me examine her eyes at length.

She agreed to fly in because, she said, "You sound friendly but realistic, like Dr. Marcus Welby on TV."

It was flattering and made me chuckle because I do not pattern myself after TV doctors. But if this is the role model that people measure their physicians by, perhaps it might be a good idea if we were all a little bit like Dr. Marcus Welby.

Mrs. Baker came in. I examined her and confirmed the fact that she had a traumatic cataract and that her right eye could and should be operated on at once. She was eager to have a permanent lens implant, and I told her that I could find no reason why it could not be done.

Right after surgery, she was able to see for several blocks outside the window and was delighted with the return of her sight.

She had been terribly fearful that the automobile accident was going to leave her totally blind. Two years had gone by since she was able to do the fine work necessary for her occupation.

"You just don't know how wonderful it is unless you haven't been able to see," she told me when she returned for a final check-up.

I have related this story so that you should know that traumatic cataracts are treated no differently than the usual cataract.

There is a lot of confusion as to whether people who suffer from cataracts of any kind and who elect lens implants ever have to wear eyeglasses. The answer to that depends on what the original lens, the one clouded by a cataract, was capable of before it became clouded.

Mrs. Baker, for example, was perfectly able to see everything without using eyeglasses, just as she had been able to do before she had the cataract. But she wore ordinary eyeglasses with prescription lenses for close work.

In other words, if you had to wear eyeglasses to correct nearsightedness or farsightedness before you had a cataract, you will generally have to wear them again after having a lens implant.

There is a very simple reason for this. The new artificial lens is matched to the clouded lens it replaces. If your original lens was such that it made you farsighted, the new lens will do the same. If your original lens was such that it made you nearsighted, the new lens will do the same. You can get back only what you had to begin with.

The same rule applies if you choose contact lenses. If you were farsighted before you had a cataract, for example, the contact lens will restore your vision to what it was; you will see clearly but will be farsighted. And you will very likely need ordinary corrective eyeglasses to enable you to read, just as you did before you had the cataract.

Similarly, the same rule applies if you choose cataract spectacles. The correction is built in.

Some people even require bifocals, just as they did before they had a cataract. Putting it simply, the vision you had before the cataract is the vision you get back.

Now I can almost hear some of you saying, "Ah, but I know people who've had cataracts taken out, and they see everything perfectly without implants, contacts, glasses, or anything!"

You are quite right. There are such fortunate people. These are people who are extremely nearsighted. Probably from the time they were quite young, they had to wear rather strong eyeglasses with perhaps a correction of –12 diopters, a measurement of extreme near-sightedness. Their original natural lens required that degree of correction.

If that lens, when clouded by a cataract, is removed, it would be ridiculous to replace it with an implant, for then they would again need corrective eyeglasses of –12 power. Incidentally, this is a glass that is thin in the middle and quite thick on the edges; a farsighted glass is just the reverse.

The mere removal of the cataract in such a patient can restore normal vision.

I must admit that this is an oversimplification of what happens, but I think it is sufficient to explain why some people do not require any kind of lens after cataract surgery. The cornea, for example, has a lot to do with the ability of the eye to focus, but I do not feel it necessary to burden you with such detail.

I think you will be served better by a real-life story, pulled from my patient file, about Sister Amanda Escontria, whose lifelong devotion to the church was threatened by her growing inability to see because of cataracts.

She was in good health despite her 84 years but was virtually blind from cataracts in both eyes, in her case a natural consequence of aging. She suffered from the kind of severe myopia—nearsightedness—that I just discussed.

Other doctors had refused to operate for fear that conventional surgery might lead to complications such as a detached retina. Using the ultrasound procedure, I saw less reason to expect any such complication, for her eyes would not be so disturbed.

I operated first on one eye and then, six months later, on the other, allowing this amount of time because of her advanced age. Both proved successful, and Sister Amanda had no need of corrective glasses to read her hymn book again. This was a direct result of the shape of the original lenses in her eyes before they became clouded by cataracts.

I am often asked, "Do most people with developing cataracts complain that their eyeglasses are not helping them see clearly?"

My answer to that question is, "Yes, many do."

But no matter whether you are nearsighted or farsighted, this has nothing to do with the development of a cataract. A cataract is not a result of any such deficiency. Neither farsightedness nor nearsightedness makes you more, or less, vulnerable. So let us put that myth to rest immediately.

I would like to go on to another very special kind of cataract called a brunescent, or brown, cataract. This is one that has really gone the distance; the heart of that clouded lens is very hard.

To remove it, the ultrasound must be modified because the heart of that cataract, what is known as the nucleus, is so hard. Too much ultrasound would be needed to vibrate that tough nucleus into liquid form.

In such cases, I would make a slightly larger incision to get at that nucleus and then dissolve the rest of the cataract with ultrasound. I could still implant an artificial lens without destroying those sturdy ligaments that hold the lens capsule in place.

I think I should mention here still another type of cataract, called a "sugar cataract," which occurs chiefly in young people and is presumably brought on by diabetes. It is uncommon, but it does occur, and blood sugar checkups are no clue to its development. However, there is no need for panic. It can be taken care of.

I have taken the trouble to mention here cataracts that differ from the usual, more common variety only because I think it important to take note of their existence and to make clear that even these are eminently curable. These special kinds of cataracts are rarely, if ever, mentioned in articles about cataracts and so often come as a stunning—in the literal sense of the word—surprise to those who suffer from them.

Now I want to speak particularly to the parents whose children have cataracts and who I know from experience are very much frightened when they are so advised.

In the fourth chapter of this book, I told you about a child who had congenital cataracts and was successfully treated. In the second chapter, I mentioned that the muscle of the eye's lens is more flexible in one's younger years. Even more importantly, you may recall that in the third chapter I talked about the need to do cataract surgery on a child before the age of six to prevent a condition known as "lazy eye," or amblyopia.

Childhood cataracts are very special. Not only must the doctor take into consideration the age of the child but also that youngster's emotional state, and the emotional state of his or her parents.

I would like to take a moment to discuss these emotional factors. If you bring a small child to see an eye specialist, that doctor must take time to talk over the whole aspect of the problem with the parents. In the case of a teen-ager, the doctor should talk directly to the youngster, just as he would to an adult.

This is just as important a part of medical care as is the operative procedure itself. It is something that family physicians are trained to comprehend but unfortunately all too many specialists overlook.

If your doctor does not take the time to discuss with you what the problem is and what is needed, medically, to overcome it, you are likely to remain afraid. I think it is most important to dispense with this fear before suggesting any medical procedure.

I want to reiterate something I said earlier about congenital cataracts, that they must be corrected before the child is 6 years old. This is very important. When a child's eye cannot see because of a cataract, it cannot be used. If it is not used, it just sits there. Without use, the eye becomes "lazy," developing the condition known as amblyopia.

You can see signs of this happening. Your child may have a habit of covering the eye to see better with the other eye, or he may keep tilting his head away from the bad eye or keep trying to brush away the blurred image in that eye.

By about the age of 6, that lazy eye could be permanently affected, and that is why I stress the need to do something about it before such time.

If cataracts of the congenital sort affect both eyes equally, then the problem is different. With such binocular cataracts, as they are called, both eyes are similarly affected, so that there is no danger of amblyopia developing.

In any case, I absolutely recommend ultrasound surgery for children, sometimes along with artificial lens implants. With rare exceptions, contact lenses are difficult for most children. The child rubs the eye, and the contact lens comes out. Then the parent has to put it in again.

Teen-agers are something else. They can handle contacts well. I would never do the conventional, old-fashioned procedure on a teen-ager because those ligaments that hold the clouded lens are just too strong to manage the traditional way. I would be fearful of pulling out more than the cataractous lens using that kind of surgical procedure.

I would not hesitate to replace that clouded lens with an artificial lens implant in a young person, but I would do so only in conjunction with the ultrasound procedure. I would want to preserve those tough ligaments, set the implant in the part of the capsule left intact, and in no way want to depend on hanging it on to the iris with sutures.

Now let me try to set aside another misconception about cataract surgery on children, that the cataract can "grow back."

A cataract, properly removed, does not and cannot grow back. When it is called a "secondary" cataract, or an "after-cataract" (most particularly in regard to adult patients), it is only a "polite" way of saying that pieces of the cataract have been left behind and have congealed into a membranous substance.

Yes, it can be corrected with another operative procedure, known as "needling," but it is not because the cataract has grown back. And I do not think you should be misled by medical euphemisms.

When anything is left in the eye, it is apt to cause inflammation and build up a membrane, but that is not a cataract even though it interferes with vision. It is easy to repair by making a slight opening in the membrane, and it is even possible to insert an artificial lens at that time, utilizing the membrane to hold it permanently in place.

I have performed such surgery many times in patients of all ages. Sometimes I encountered situations in which it was necessary to improvise such a surgical procedure on the spot.

In one case, involving an 8-year-old youngster named Ilmar Suazo, who was flown in from the Dominican Republic, I developed a procedure that I called "drumstick surgery."

What had happened was that Ilmar's congenital cataracts had been operated on by conventional surgery, but almost three-fourths of the cataract material had been left in the child's eyes. This material had formed a thickened membrane that left the child blind, and the parents were frantic.

When I looked into Ilmar's eyes through the operating microscope, the membrane had the appearance of a tightened drumskin. It was so thick that simply making a hole in it would not be sufficient, for that hole would quickly seal over, and the problem would remain.

There was only one way to correct the problem. I had to use two scalpels, working them like drumsticks against the thickened membrane to make a permanent opening so that Ilmar could see again.

The procedure took but five minutes. By the following day, sufficient healing had taken place for Ilmar to see again. His mother was ecstatic and called it a miracle. But it was not a miracle. Any experienced cataract surgeon could have performed the same or similar procedure.

I have brought up this case merely to indicate that even when things go wrong, the problem is usually reversible. Even an implant placed in the eye by the conventional procedure can be removed and replaced if necessary in most cases, though this is a problem that occurs rarely and just about never with ultrasound.

The whole point that I want to make here is that you do frequently have a second chance in those uncommon instances in which the final results are less than you expected. Few operative procedures can make this claim.

I make this point only to reassure readers whose fear of cataract surgery is so great that it produces all sorts of far-out possibilities of risk.

Do not misunderstand me. There can be complications, but the possibility of such is nearly always evident before the operation. For example, say that you have glaucoma. If it is not under control, you should not undergo cataract surgery by any method. However, if it is under control, I would not hesitate to use the ultrasound procedure.

The same applies if you have hypertension, if it

is controlled. In both situations, you could have a lens implant.

If you are diabetic, I would want to know if your retina is affected and how healthy your iris is. If you suffer from diabetic retinopathy (leaking blood vessels in the retina) or have an inflamed iris, I would take every precaution before recommending cataract surgery, but chances are good that you would be able to do so if your other problem is treated simultaneously. I may not, however, give you an implant.

You may have heard some talk about corneal edema (swelling of the cornea) following a lens implant. This can result from damage to the cells inside the cornea. Since the ultrasound procedure is far less disturbing to the eye, there is little chance of this happening. As a matter of fact, I have never had a single patient suffer from corneal edema among the more than a thousand lens implants I have done.

I would advise you to have an implant inserted at the time you have the cataract removed, not afterward. Oh, it can be done even afterward with the ultrasound procedure, because the ligaments are not disturbed, and part of the lens capsule is still there to hold the artificial lens. But it does mean having to open the eye twice. So, clearly, it is more sensible to do both procedures simultaneously: removal of the cataract and insertion of the artificial lens.

One final point. Cataract patients sometimes say that their eye looks different after their operation, that the pupil does not look quite the same. This is usually because they have undergone the old-fashioned procedure and a piece of the iris was taken out, sometimes in the shape of a keyhole, to make the clouded cataract lens more accessible. This is unnecessary with the ultrasound procedure.

The important thing for the cataract patient is to have confidence in the surgeon he or she selects and to be familiar with the procedure that surgeon practices. The key word here is skill, and there are ways to estimate it so that you can make a truly informed decision.

VIII

How to Find the Right Doctor

In the very first chapter of this book, I made it clear that I agreed with those of my professional colleagues who feel that a cataract surgeon should be able to do all types of cataract operations.

I make no secret of the fact that I favor the ultrasound procedure in almost every case. But on those rare occasions when the conventional procedure is necessary or when the ultrasound procedure has to be modified, I am prepared to adjust.

So, too, should the eye surgeon you select.

Even beyond all other considerations, be absolutely certain that the surgeon you select will operate, not merely oversee it. Like me, he may have other doctors working under his supervision, but I would strongly suggest that you apply to the doctor you consult the same rule that you would apply if you consulted me.

You would want me to operate, and that is who you would get. I do all the cataract surgery in Germantown Hospital, in Philadelphia.

You should expect as much from the doctor you consult.

Why? Because one of the most important requirements for a cataract surgeon is experience—good, successful experience. There must be skill to start with, and there must be continued experience to sharpen that skill.

Cataract surgery should present no surprises to the doctor.

The doctor you choose should of course possess steady hands, fine coordination, and be thoroughly familiar with the operating microscope.

And he should have lots and lots of practice.

I deliberately elect to do some 20 cataract procedures each week to maintain my skills. To do less over a period of time would tend to diminish those skills; to do more would tend to push me beyond my natural capacity.

I am talking here not only about removing the cataract but also about implanting an artificial lens. Because both go hand in hand. I want always to be as familiar with one as with the other.

So when you consult an ophthalmologist about a cataract, be sure to ask not only how many operations he has done, but also how often he does them, week in and week out.

Be realistic. You would not want to undergo open-heart surgery, for example, by a heart surgeon with a flimsy or off-again, on-again track record, would you?

Granted, cataract surgery is by no means in the same league, surgically speaking, as heart surgery, but it is for you.

Because you want to be sure, you want to have absolute confidence in your doctor and in his technique.

It is for this very reason that some hospitals were not granted official professional approval for heart surgery; the cardiac surgeons at those hospitals were insufficiently practiced in such operations.

Be equally circumspect when choosing a doctor to remove a cataract from your eye. Know precisely the extent of his experience in order to have full confidence in him.

I consider it a doctor's obligation to place his patient's welfare ahead of everything else, and this includes keeping up with the lastest developments in his field.

When a new, safe, fully-approved medical procedure becomes available and is shown to be more beneficial than the old tried-and-true methods, that doctor should be ready to employ it in his practice.

If I were a cataract patient, this is the only kind of doctor in whom I would place my trust. For I would feel confident that he knew all there is to know about his special field and that he knew it not only from his readings but from his actual experience in the operating room.

Remember what I said earlier about a cataract surgeon's needing to be familiar with all types of operations? And with lens implant procedures?

Well, this is what it is all about when it comes to finding the right doctor to take care of your cataract.

Almost 20 percent of all cataract surgery done these days is handled by the ultrasound procedure, and almost 10 percent involve a lens implant as well.

The percentages should be greater. All of the professional data bear this out. Let me cite some examples.

The National Aeronautics and Space Administration (NASA) has made the medical profession aware of this in a recent news release.

NASA states very clearly:

> A cataract is a condition in which the lens of the eye becomes opaque, impairing vision and leading to potential blindness. Surgery to remove the cloudy material is necessary to restore vision. About half a million people a year need such surgery in the United States alone. Traditional surgical techniques require a 180-degree incision and then numerous stitches to close it and the possibility of infection keeps patients in the hospital for at least a 10-day recovery period.

So we are talking about the need for what some people like to refer to as "space-age surgery," and that is what ultrasound is all about.

But let me go on. The *FDA Consumer,* a journal of the U.S. government published in the public interest, has this to say about implant surgery: "The most common problem with new implants is that they can become dislocated in the eye. This can happen to the clip-on type when the iris becomes too widely dilated, permitting the lens to slip back through the pupil."

And that is the way lens implants are put in with the old-fashioned, conventional procedure. It is not the way implants are put in with the ultrasound procedure.

Why do I tell you all this?

Because I want you to know that the ultrasound procedure is not only fully accepted professionally but also offers the cataract patient a great many advantages. And it is important that your doctor be thoroughly conversant with this procedure, no less than he is with the old-fashioned way of treating cataracts.

You may have to shop around a bit until you find a doctor familiar with and capable of all approaches to cataract surgery, including lens implantation.

This was the case with a patient of mine named Mrs. Helen Mamoudis. Her cataracts had progressed to the point at which she was unable to see her fingers in front of her right eye.

She had visited an eye doctor who was totally unfamiliar with ultrasound and, for that reason, was dead set against it. But Mrs. Mamoudis had heard about ultrasound and was not satisfied with that kind of appraisal.

Somehow or other, she had heard about the work I am doing with ultrasound and lens implants and decided to consult me about her problem.

What I found was that her left eye was strained due to the cataract in her right eye. It was no wonder that she was unable to see well even directly in front of her.

I was forced to take issue with the ophthalmologist who had examined her and to explain to her that she would not have to undergo prolonged hospitalization to regain her vision. Nor did I agree with him that she would have to wear cataract spectacles. An implant was definitely indicated and would make spectacles unnecessary.

She was convinced by my explanation, and I did the required procedure, implanting a new lens in her right eye. She was delighted with the result and attended a political convention two days after the operation. Her vision was perfect.

"I believe I would have gone blind if I had not found this way of treating my cataract," she told me.

What impressed her particularly is that she experienced no pain during or after the procedure. "I've had no problems," she told me. "There's been no need for pain medicine of any kind."

However, she was upset by the diagnosis of the doctor she had consulted earlier and the treatment he had recommended. Being something of a political person, Mrs. Mamoudis was all gung-ho to go to Washington and tell the Congress of her experience.

"I'd like to go to Washington and show some of those old birds with their specs," she said. "I'd take away their glasses and see if they could see as well as I do!"

I relate this story only to make plain to my readers that the ultrasound procedure, phacoemulsification, is not a procedure with which every eye specialist is familiar, but I think it is important that he should be. The same goes for lens implantation.

Hardly a day goes by when I do not see patients who have had conventional cataract surgery in one eye and pretty good vision in the other eye so that they do not need surgery there. But they have to wear a contact lens in the operated eye and just cannot handle it. Without it, they have double vision. That could be worse than having had no cataract surgery at all.

Eye doctors must make this possibility clear to their patients before they operate.

When I see a patient, I show them a model of their eye, point out where the lens is that is clouded by a cataract, and explain why it must come out and how it can be replaced.

I consider it not only a medical but also a legal responsibility to do so. It is very unfortunate that some cataract surgeons who do not do implants never bother to mention that here is another way to correct vision after surgery.

Even more appalling to me, judging from the comments of my patients, is that some eye surgeons do not bother to mention at all that some kind of replacement lens, some kind of substitute lens, will be needed after surgery. Then, quite suddenly after surgery, the patient is shocked to learn that he or she will have to wear cataract spectacles or contact lenses.

I have had patient after patient complain to me that this is what happened after cataract surgery on one eye and that they complained to the doctor, "But I can't stand contact lenses, and I really don't want cataract spectacles even if they help me to see better." And they are told, "Well, you will have to wear a contact lens. That is the only way you will be able to see again."

This could be torture to the person who cannot handle a contact lens, particularly an elderly person in whom the success rate with contact lenses is no more than 50 percent.

In some cases, it is even better for the cataract to remain if the other eye is good; at least these people would be able to see normally through that one good eye without having to endure double vision due to their inability to use a contact lens in the operated eye.

Unfortunately, you cannot test a contact lens beforehand. You can make an educated guess as to a person's ability to handle the insertion and extraction of a contact lens and to some extent size up the eye: how much it tends to tearing, how droopy the lids may be, whether or not there is conjunctivitis of a chronic kind, or corneal distortion or some kind of allergy.

But the cataract patient who chooses to wear a contact lens must not only be able to do so in regard to the way the eye is structured but also must be attuned to it psychologically. In short, the ideal contact lens patient must be motivated to go to the trouble necessary to wear that contact lens, if not of the hard variety, then of the soft kind.

But this is something that must be discussed before cataract surgery.

The alternative of an artificial lens implant should be made clear before any surgery is done.

There are people, for example, who could not tolerate contact lenses long before they had cataracts. So there is no reason to suspect that they would be able to tolerate them, as they must, after cataract surgery. I would never contemplate surgery on such people without talking to them about their considering lens implants, which would do away with the need for contact lenses.

Despite the high success rate of cataract surgery, it is not a frivolous procedure. And it must be considered in terms of the individual patient.

Furthermore, if I were a cataract patient, I would want to know which procedure had the least possible complications. That would have to be the ultrasound procedure, done routinely by a doctor well versed in it, because there is less trauma to the eye with ultrasound, a far smaller incision, and much less disturbance to the structure of the eye.

And I would willingly sign a consent form, as I ask my patients to do, to the effect that, as my consent form puts it: "The procedures necessary to remedy my condition have been explained to me by the surgeon and I understand the nature of the surgery to be as represented."

I would expect that my doctor would be familiar with all types of cataract surgery and with lens implants.

Well, finding such a doctor is not always easy. All ophthalmologists are not conversant with the phacoemulsification procedure that I have referred to as ultrasound. Fewer still are familiar with lens implants, and even fewer are proficient at both ultrasound and lens-implant techniques.

So, you may have to do some looking about if you have a cataract. And I would certainly advise you to do so.

Ultrasound surgery does require specialized training in the use of the ultrasonic probe and the operating microscope. Older surgeons who have performed thousands of successful operations with the old-fashioned procedure often see no reason to learn the newer method. Some, in fact, are no longer steady enough to master the newer technique.

Still, I believe that they should make it plain to you that newer methods are available to cure cataracts and that they offer many advantages to you, the patient.

If you are not given such information, you cannot make a truly informed decision. While I believe that every cataract patient should rely on the judgment of his or her ophthalmologist as to when and what type of surgery is needed, I do not believe that such advice should be offered without an awareness of all that is happening in the field of cataract surgery.

Fortunately, nearly all eye surgeons are today aware of advances in cataract surgery, and that includes a knowledge of the ultrasound procedure and lens implantation. But many, for reasons that I will go into later, do not or cannot perform either the ultrasound procedure or the implant procedure.

Let me sum up the chapter in this way. If you have a cataract and are searching for the right doctor to take care of it, do the following:

1. Ask your family doctor to recommend someone.
2. Talk to friends who have had cataract surgery.
3. Ask the doctor you consult how many cataract operations and implants he does each week.
4. Ask him if he does ultrasound surgery, how long he has been doing it, and if he uses it only on certain cases.
5. Ask him what sort of corrective lenses you will need after surgery.
6. Ask him how long you will be incapacitated before regaining your sight and how long you will be hospitalized.
7. And ask him his price.

Good eye doctors rarely give bad advice. But the cost of cataract surgery is something else. We will talk more about that in the next chapter.

IX

What It Costs to Cure Cataracts

If you were in my position and writing this book, I am sure that you, like me, would be very much tempted to repeat that old chestnut about not being able to put a price on "priceless sight."

But I am sure you will agree that this would be overbearing, even arrogant. And that is not my style.

Sure, sight is precious. However, that hard-earned money of yours that you have to put down to regain your sight is precious, too.

So I am going to talk about those costs here within those limits that the ethics of my profession allow, and those are broad enough to allow me to be sufficiently specific.

No matter what your financial situation might be, I am certain that you will feel more comfortable knowing what everything costs and how those costs can be met.

Just remember that cataract surgery is a big business. Three out of four eye operations are for cataracts. This is not intended to suggest in any way that eye surgeons are out to "rip you off." Not by any means. My only purpose in making that statement is to advise you that there is more to cataract surgery than meets the eye, no pun intended.

There is politics in eye care just as there is in every other area of life.

All cataract surgeons, and they include me, love cataract surgery, not simply because it is a way of making a living, but because it is one of the most satisfying and successful surgical procedures in all of medicine.

It does wonders for me professionally when I am able to restore someone's sight. It also does wonders for my ego; oh, yes, no doubt about it. If it seems like something miraculous to my patient, it seems something like that to me as well, no matter how many times I have done the same procedure.

Don't ever underestimate a doctor's ego!

Still, it is this need for success that makes a doctor a good doctor.

Unfortunately, it is also why some doctors hesitate to master newer techniques, such as the ultrasound procedure. They are good doctors, and they know how to eliminate cataracts. Many have performed thousands of cataract operations using the old-fashioned procedure and see no reason why they should change now and augment their skills by becoming adept at the ultrasound procedure as well as the conventional method to which they are accustomed.

Older surgeons may no longer possess the kind of manual dexterity and coordination needed to use ultrasound to remove a cataract or implant an artificial lens. This is why you will find that most ultrasound eye surgeons are on the young side.

So do not be too surprised if the highly reputable eye doctor you consult does not recommend the ultrasound procedure or even a lens implant. In all likelihood, he has not mastered these techniques.

This is why I use the word "politics." The ultrasound procedure has full medical accreditation, and the doctor you consult about your cataract should be able to use it just as easily as he can use the old-fashioned method.

But there is another political aspect to eye surgery.

The traditional operation can be performed in any hospital. The ultrasound procedure requires a lot of very special expensive equipment. The computerized ultrasound equipment alone requires an expense of at least $25,000. The operating microscope costs about $20,000. And all these costs are rising, as are all hospital expenditures.

This is one reason why many hospital administrators are less than enthusiastic about ultrasound. There is another reason, and that has to do with the fact that hospital beds are occupied for long periods by cataract patients who have undergone traditional surgery.

Short hospital stays, or none at all, are not as advantageous financially as are longer hospital stays.

That is what I call political expedience.

But it is at your expense, for you are the patient. And every eye surgeon and all hospitals are well aware that ultrasound is an accepted and approved procedure.

Every medical policy written will help pay for it. So, too, will Medicare. These are called third-party payments, meaning that somebody else helps you pay the doctor and, if required, the hospital bill as well.

What does all this add up to in dollars and cents?

The surgeon's fee is the same as for the ordinary procedure and could range from as little as $750 to as high as $2,500, the higher fee generally including the implant procedure as well. These fees reflect, to some extent, the reputation of the surgeon and the city in which he practices. Surgeons in some large cities may charge higher fees because their own expenses are higher in those areas.

If hospitalization is required, this adds to the cost, and it could be considerable. The usual hospitalization period for the old-fashioned procedure is 5–10 days. With the way hospital costs keep rising, this expense could run to several thousand dollars.

If you require cataract spectacles following surgery, you can figure on spending about $200. A single contact lens can cost about $150. Bear in mind, too, that both cataract glasses and contact lenses frequently need to be replaced because of loss, breakage, or a possible change in the prescription.

The artificial implant is absolutely the least expensive type of replacement lens. Its cost is about $150, but unlike cataract glasses or contact lenses, the implant is permanent and never needs replacing.

With Blue Cross, Medicare, or other major medical insurance, these expenses will be greatly diminished and perhaps even eliminated entirely. Even the cost of an implant is generally absorbed by your health insurance coverage, just as it would cover you for, say, a cardiac pacemaker or a hip prosthesis.

If you do not carry such insurance and have to pay your own way, your total cost could add up to quite a lot of money. But even if you are covered by insurance that will pay part, or even most, of your total bill, you should consider something else by which to measure the cost of correcting your cataract problem.

Do you really want to stay in a hospital for several days or even weeks? Can you afford to miss going back to work? Are you willing to stretch out the amount of time needed to recover from cataract surgery?

If your answer to these questions is "No," then you should definitely consider having your cataract removed by the ultrasound procedure. I have already discussed at some length the advantages of this procedure, so I am not going to bother going into it again. I merely want to impress on you the importance of consulting a surgeon who is experienced in *all* types of cataract procedures so that you can make a truly informed decision.

This may necessitate your visiting a second surgeon to obtain a second opinion. Do so. If you have a medical policy, it will most likely cover the added expense. Getting this second opinion will do a lot for your peace of mind.

It does not offend me if a patient asks to seek a second opinion before choosing me as his or her surgeon. In fact, I encourage it. And I see no reason why any doctor should feel offended.

Moreover, if a patient cannot meet my fee and has no recourse to third-party payment, I will not let the lack of money stand in the way of treatment. No doctor should do less.

But keep in mind that the cost of regaining good sight must be measured not only in dollars. I told you in the first chapter of this book about a man named Stanley Wallace whose both eyes were clouded by cataracts. After the ultrasound procedure had removed both cataracts, he told me, "That older type of operation would have kept me from work and, in the long run, would have cost a lot more."

The same goes for Mr. Richard Dempsey and Mr. Ted Hoeger, whom I have told you about earlier. These were businessmen who had to get back to work as quickly as possible.

And lest you think I am being "sexist," let me refer you back to the previous chapter in this book and the case of Mrs. Helen Mamoudis. She wasted no time getting back to business following cataract surgery with the ultrasound procedure, having rejected the possibility of similar surgery by the old-fashioned method, which would have meant prolonged inactivity.

"I just dropped that idea altogether," she told me.

To put it briefly, the cost of cataract surgery is relative not only to your ability to pay, or even to the extent of your medical-insurance coverage, but also to the degree of inconvenience and discomfort you are willing to put up with and to the amount of time you are able to spend recovering from the operation.

All of these elements should be taken into consideration by the individual contemplating cataract surgery, along with the doctor's reputation, his track record in such procedures, and the recommendations of friends or family physicians.

Take all of these elements into account beforehand not only to keep down the financial expense but also to alleviate the psychological burden.

X

Why You Should Stop Worrying

Surely, if you have read this far, I hope that by now you have laid aside whatever fears you had of cataracts. You know how the ultrasound procedure, and even the old-fashioned operation, can render you free of cataracts and restore your vision. You know, too, that medical science has perfected an artificial lens that fits inside your eye to replace that clouded lens for all time.

Worry about losing one's sight is very understandable. Almost everyone has had the awful experience of having something in their eye, and even though that may steal away their sight for no more than a brief few minutes, it arouses panic. Moreover, blindness—unlike cancer or heart disease, for example—is something you can see in

the individual who must use a cane to tap-tap-tap his way across the street or hold fast to a seeing-eye dog.

You cannot so easily see the ravages of cancer or the anxiousness in heart patients. But the effects of blindness, ironically, are plainly visible to the sighted.

I think this has a lot to do with the fear such a disability arouses not only among those with good vision but also, and most particularly, among those whose cataracts are stealthily robbing them of good vision.

Is it not a great relief to know that now you can put such worries out of your mind once and for all?

Forget about all those old wives' tales you may have heard about cataracts, like smearing honey or cow dung on your eyelids to cure them, or reaching out in desperation for some vitamin or special diet to get rid of them.

The only way to be rid of a cataract is by a simple, pain-free operative procedure. And now the benefits of ultrasound, often in conjunction with a permanent lens implant, make available a revolutionary approach to curing cataracts that several hundred thousand persons have already enjoyed.

"Now that the computer-monitored instrument for phacoemulsification (ultrasound) has been improved," comments a professional publication addressed to physicians and eye surgeons in training, "it seems probable that this procedure will be used by more ophthalmic surgeons familiar with microsurgery."

The key word there to keep in mind is "familiar," meaning that the eye surgeon has great expertise in this procedure, uses it regularly week in and week out, and prefers it over any other.

It is not enough for you to know the total number of ultrasound procedures and lens implants he has done. You should ask how many he does each week. When I am asked, my answer is, "I do twenty such procedures each week. All in all, I've done more than three thousand ultrasound procedures successfully and more than one thousand lens implants." Every doctor should be equally specific.

You ought not to select a cataract surgeon for convenience' sake, because his office or hospital is just around the corner from your home. Traveling even to another city is surely worth the extra expense if it means getting the best treatment for your eyes. It no longer surprises me to see patients, some of whom you have read about in this book, who have come from clear across the country and even from abroad.

Incidentally, a question that is often put to me is, "Tell me, Dr. Brooks, what will happen if I should be hit in the eye, and I have an implant?"

My answer is, "If you had the old-fashioned operation using clips and sutures, there's a greater chance that the lens will come loose. But with ultrasound and the lens supported by the natural capsule in your eye, that lens is just as firmly attached as the human lens. That human lens could come loose if you have an accident, but that shouldn't stop you from playing impact sports, for example. Well, you can't do that if you had the standard operation with an implant, but you can with the ultrasound procedure. And you could do it a lot more safely than if you were wearing a contact lens that could damage your cornea."

So let us put that fear to rest.

One of the great difficulties faced by cataract patients is not having such matters explained to them by their doctors. Do you recall, for example, my having mentioned in the third chapter of this book the case of an airline pilot whose vision was still extremely good despite a progressive cataract but not good enough to permit him to keep flying?

He had 20/25 vision, but he needed 20/20. I would never dream of doing such a delicate procedure any other way than with the ultrasound technique. It was not a matter of heading off blindness but of refining the man's vision to make it flawless again. Well, after the healing process, his cornea regained its normal curvature again, and his 20/20 vision returned. He was able to resume his flight duties.

That is an extreme case. Now here is another extreme case, of quite a different kind, about a delightful lady of 82 who called herself "the six-million dollar grandma" because she already had an artificial hip, a cardiac pacemaker, and—following ultrasound surgery—a lens implant.

"Now I've even got a bionic eye," she told me,

"and I can see and read again for the first time in over a year."

Between these two extremes is a middle-aged gentleman named Mr. Orville Gardner. He had hunted high and low for a doctor who could do the ultrasound procedure because he wanted a choice before deciding on cataract surgery. Unable to find one in his area, he and his wife flew in to consult with me at Germantown Hospital, traveling all the way from Michigan to Philadelphia.

He decided on ultrasound and an implant and was very happy with the result. "We'd like to tell others about our experience," he said to me afterward, "because people should have a choice if they have cataracts. Doctors aren't telling people about the new procedure, and the old technique is leaving many older persons we know virtually crippled."

Mr. Jesse Yoder, whose story I related in the second chapter of this book, explained his feelings this way. "It's remarkable the things that are happening these days," he told me. "We just go along and enjoy them. I'm glad for the improvements."

You be glad, too. Your cataracts are curable. Everyone's are. And you do have a choice.

So you can stop worrying.

INDEX